MDSAP

Vol.5 of 5 USA

For All

(Employees & Employers)

Second Edition:

Online Certification

www.silosa.ca

Jahangir Asadi

Vancouver, BC CANADA

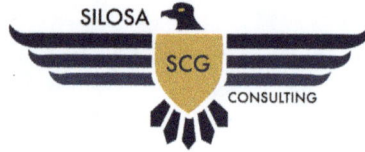

Published by: Silosa Consulting Group Inc.
Vancouver, BC **CANADA**
Email: Info@Silosa.ca
www.silosa.ca

Ordering Information:
Quantity sales. Special discounts are available on quantity purchases by universities, schools, corporations, associations, and others. For details, contact the "Sales Department" at the above mentioned email address.

MDSAP Vol.1-5 (for all employees and employers)/J.Asadi—2nd ed.
ISBN: 978-1-990451-55-3   Vol.1 Australia Paperback
ISBN: 978-1-990451-56-0   Vol.2 Brazil   Paperback
ISBN: 978-1-990451-57-7   Vol.3 Canada   Paperback
ISBN: 978-1-990451-58-4   Vol.4 Japan   Paperback
ISBN: 978-1-990451-59-1   Vol.5 USA   Paperback

Contents

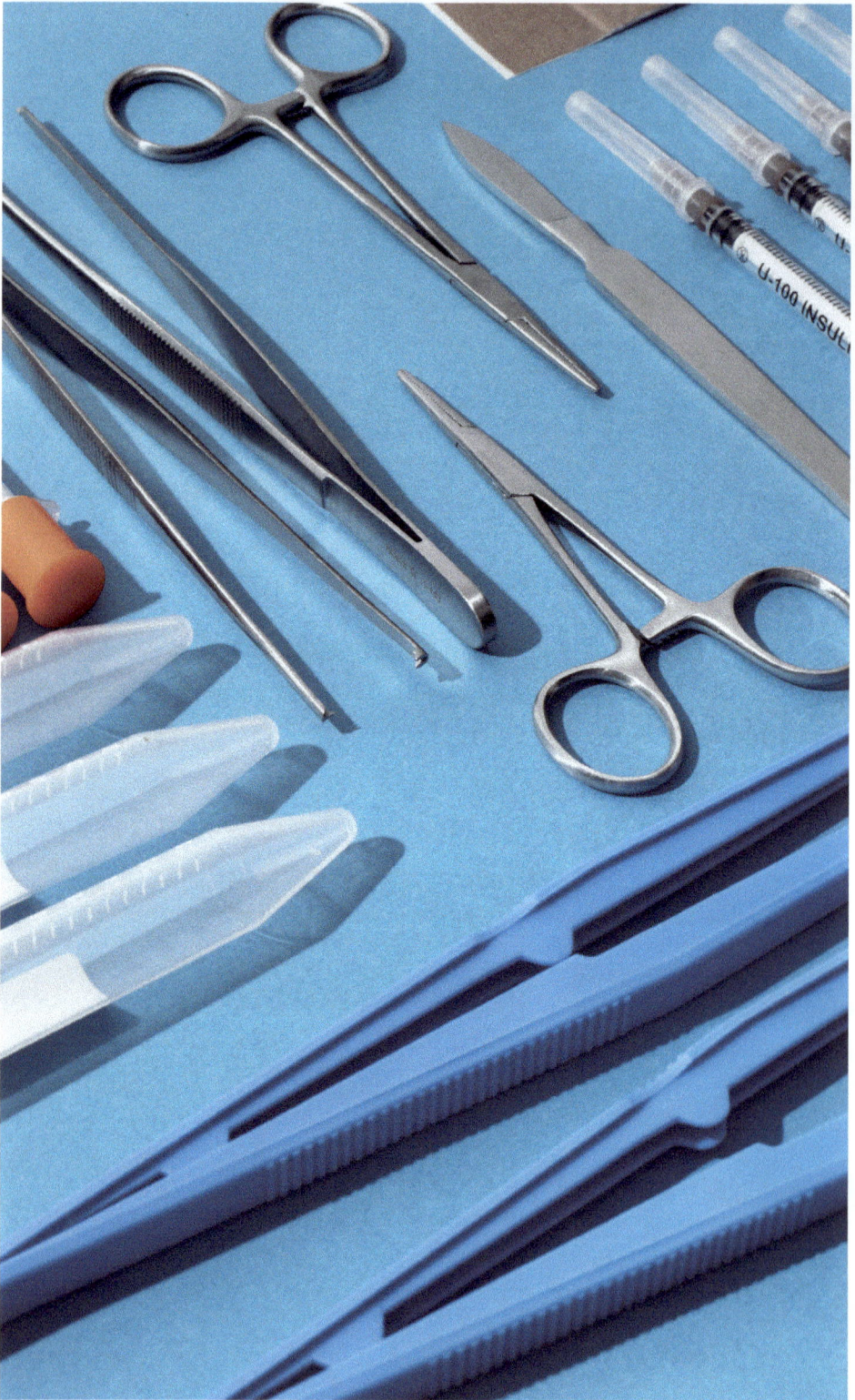

This book is dedicated to my first manager,

Mir Ahmad Sadat,

a Distinguished man of ISIRI, who has been
my supporter and has encouraged me greatly
and believed genuinely in my ability with
honesty and self-confidence.

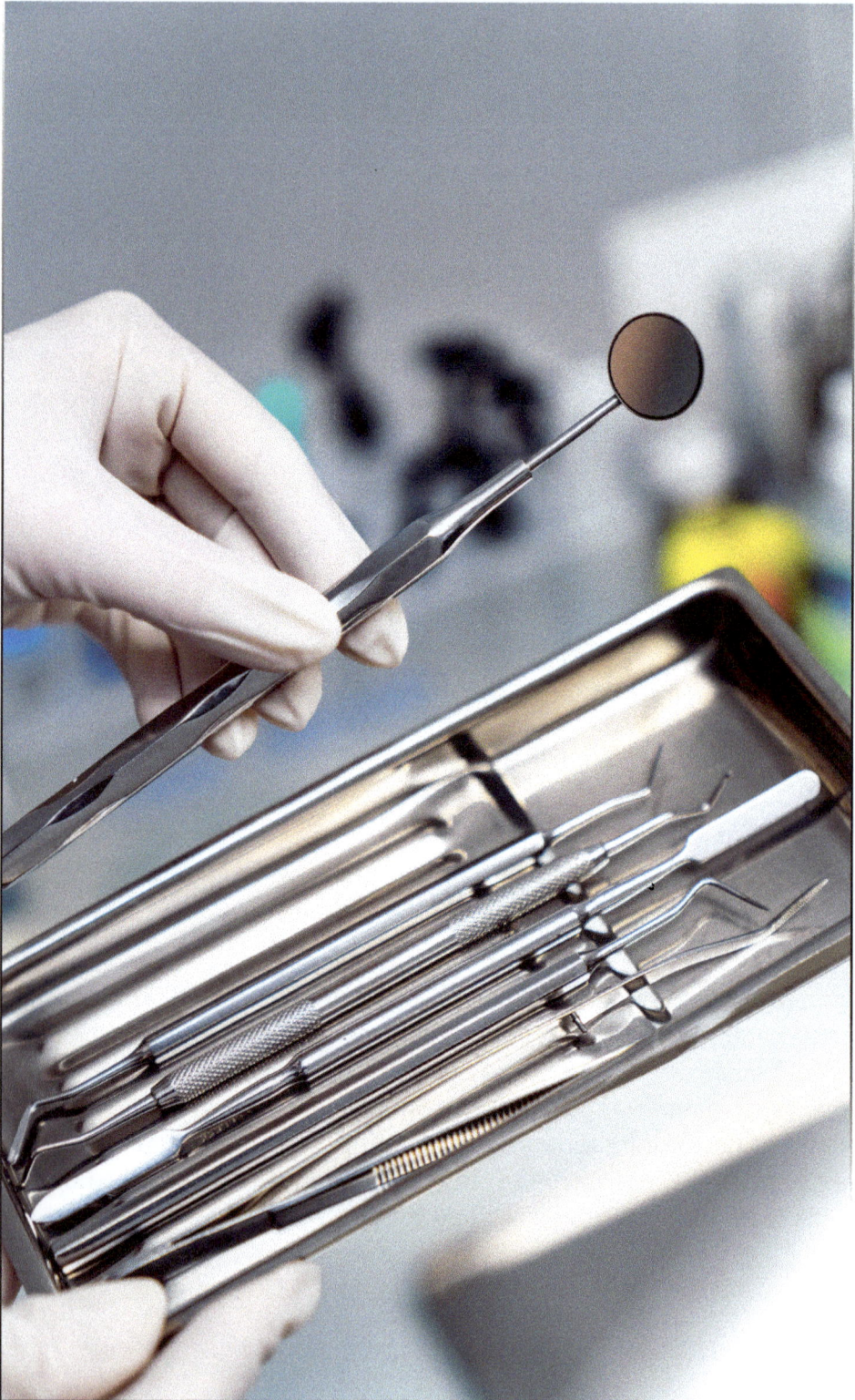

SILOSA Consulting Group (SCG)

Silosa Consulting Group (SCG) was established to provide out-standing consulting services of management system standards to individuals, groups, companies, and organizations all over the globe.

SCG is publishing an "EASY ISO" book series related to International Management System Standards to increase public knowledge in implementing these systems over their organizations.

SCG book publishing services and distribution services are connected to over 39,000 booksellers worldwide, including Apple, Amazon, Barnes & Noble, Indigo, Google Play Books, and many more. We focus on quality, environmental, food safety and other management system standards.

SCG has enough experiences to help create new and effective programmes in different countries all over the world. For more detail, visit our

website : http://silosa.ca and/or send your enquiery to the following email:

info@silosa.ca

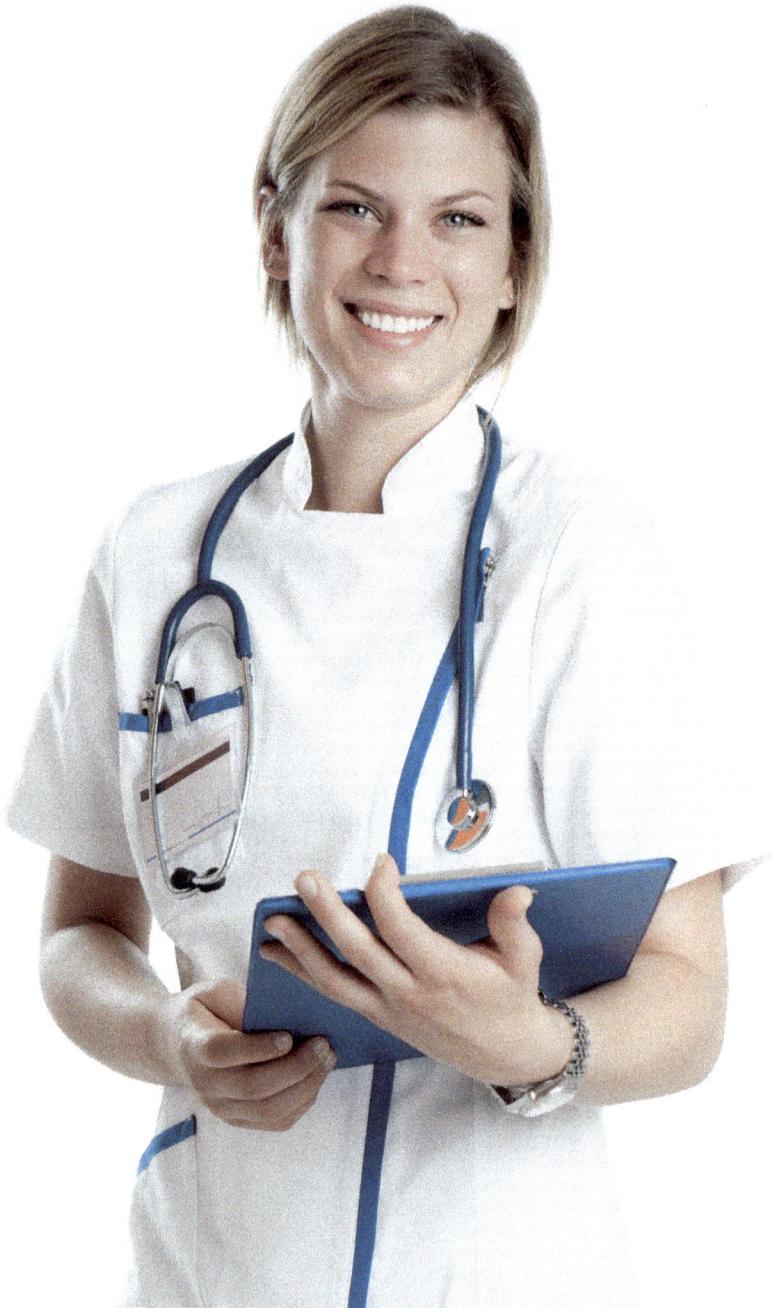

CHAPTER 1

About ISO

The International Organization for Standardization is an independent, non-governmental organization, the members of which are the standards organizations of the 165 member countries. It is the world's largest developer of voluntary international standards and it facilitates world trade by providing common standards among nations. More than twenty thousand standards have been set, covering everything from manufactured products and technology to food safety, agriculture, and healthcare.

Use of the standards aids in the creation of products and services that are safe, reliable, and of good quality. The standards help businesses increase productivity while minimizing errors and waste. By enabling products from different markets to be directly compared, they facilitate companies in entering new markets and assist in the development of global trade on a fair basis. The standards also serve to safeguard consumers and the end-users of products and services, ensuring that certified products conform to the minimum standards set internationally.

History

The organization began in the 1920s as the International Federation of the National Standardizing Associations (ISA). It was suspended in 1942 during World War II, but after the war ISA was approached by the recently formed United Nations Standards Coordinating Committee (UNSCC) with a proposal to form a new global standards body. In October 1946, ISA and UNSCC delegates from 25 countries met in London and agreed to join forces to create the new International Organization for Standardization. The new organization officially began operations in February 1947.

More information can be obtained :

www.ISO.org

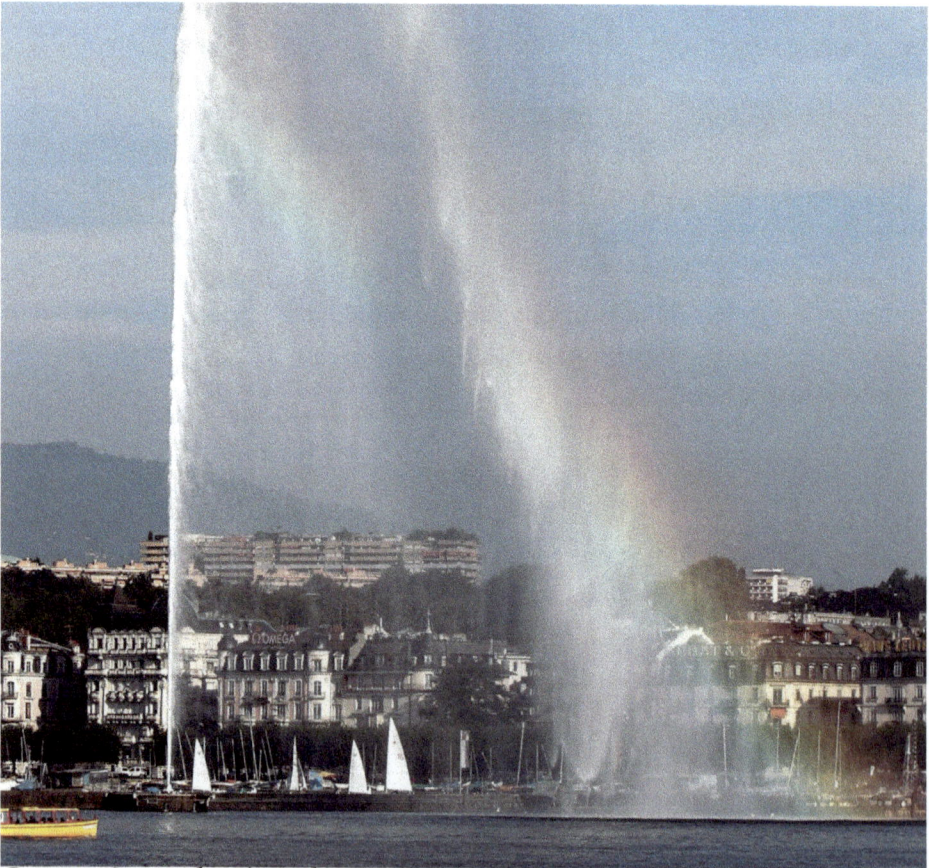

Geneva, Switzerlan (Headquarter of ISO)

CHAPTER 2

MDSAP

MDSAP The Medical Device Single Audit Program is the single audit program that covers the regulations of Australia, Brazil, Canada, Japan and USA. These regulations use the MDSAP to verify compliance to the quality systems of their national regulations and ISO 13485. The intention of the Medical Device Single Audit Program (MDSAP) is to allow competent auditors from MDSAP recognized Auditing Organizations (AOs) to conduct a single audit of a medical device organization's quality management system that will satisfy the requirements of the medical device regulatory authorities participating in the MDSAP program.

Audits performed under the MDSAP program will be process based, focusing on several defined processes, a defined method for linking those processes, and built on a foundation of requirements for risk management.

ISO 13485 MDSAP are two different programs with similar requirements but they do not duplicate each other.

MDSAP has the more stringent requirements of the two and companies that are already certified to ISO 13485 will see an increase in the number of audit days once they seek certification to MDSAP. The design of the Medical Device Single Audit Program (MDSAP) audit process is to ensure a single audit will provide efficient yet thorough coverage of regulatory requirements.

These requirements include; Medical devices – Quality management systems – Requirements for regulatory purposes (ISO 13485:2016), the Quality Management System requirements of the Conformity Assessment Procedures of the Australian Therapeutic

Goods (Medical Devices) Regulations (TG(MD)R Sch3), the Brazilian Good Manufacturing Practices (RDC ANVISA 16/2013), the Japanese Ordinance on Standards for Manufacturing Control and Quality Control of Medical Devices and In Vitro Diagnostic Reagents (MHLW Ministerial Ordinance No. 169), the Quality System Regulation (21 CFR Part 820), and specific requirements of the medical device regulatory authorities participating in the MD-SAP program.

What is the meaning of ISO 13485 certified?

ISO certification is a seal of approval from a third party body that a company runs to one of the international standards developed and published by the International Organization for Standardization (ISO). ... ISO 13485 helps put your customers first.

Is ISO 13485 certification worth it?

ISO 13485 is important to designers, manufacturers, and distributors of medical devices. In addition, suppliers and service providers can enhance an organization's marketability as more and more manufacturers require certification in order to do business with a vendor.

MDSAP AUDIT:

The design and development of the MDSAP audit sequence allows a logical, focused and efficient conduct of an audit. The MDSAP audit sequence follows a process approach and has four primary processes - Management process, Measurement, Analysis and Improvement process, Design and Development process and a Production and Service Controls process with links to the supporting process for Purchasing.

The definition of each process includes a purpose and an outcome that are indicators of process performance. Each participating Regulatory Authority expects that risk management to be the foundation for the five processes that are the requirements of a quality management system for medical device organizations.

The MDSAP audit process has two additional supporting processes: Device Marketing Authorization and Facility Registration and Medical Device Adverse Events and Advisory Notices Reporting. These processes are necessary to fulfill specific requirements of the participating MDSAP regulatory authorities.

Regulatory Requirements

Country	Regulatory	MDSAP
Australia	Conformity Assessment Procedures of the Australian Therapeutic Goods (Medical Devices) Regulations (TG(MD)R Sch3)	Vo.1
Brazil	The Brazilian Good Manufacturing Practices (RDC ANVISA 2013/16)	Vol.2
Canada	Medical Devices Regulations SOR/282-98 and specific requirements of the medical device regulatory authorities	Vol.3
Japan	The Japanese Ordinance on Standards for Manufacturing Control and Quality Control of Medical Devices and In Vitro Diagnostic Reagents (MHLW Ministerial Ordinance No. 169),	Vol.4
USA	FDA Quality System Regulation (21 CFR Part 820)	Vol.5

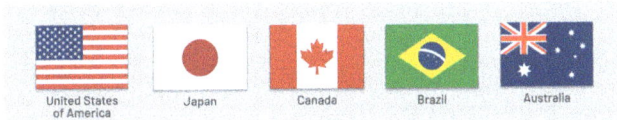

United States of America   Japan   Canada   Brazil   Australia

Definitions

ISO 13485 specifies requirements for a quality management system where an organization needs to demonstrate its ability to provide medical devices and related services that consistently meet customer and applicable regulatory requirements. Such organizations can be involved in one or more stages of the life-cycle, including design and development, production, storage and distribution, installation, or servicing of a medical device and design and development or provision of associated activities (e.g. technical support). ISO 13485 can also be used by suppliers or external parties that provide product, including quality management system-related services to such organizations.

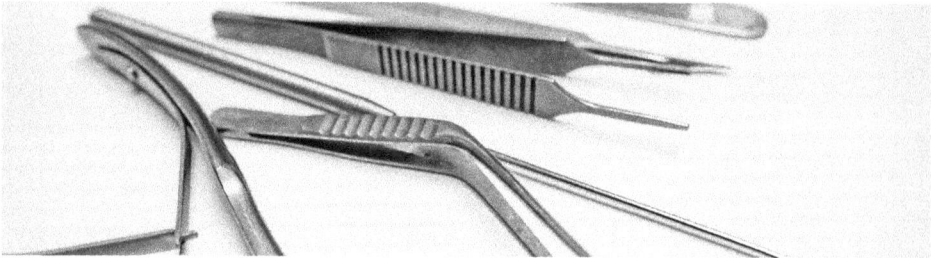

Scope of Certificate: The scope of the ISO certificate depends on how your Organization would like to have keeping in view of future. Some want to be specific by listing the products; some to be general covering the broad category of products. Here are some examples:

1. Design, development assemble, manufacture, distribute and service of life science instruments

2. Design, assemble/manufacture, sales & service of medical instruments used in cardiology including ECG Recorders, Bedside monitors

3. Design, development, manufacture, distribute and repair of medical device instruments intended to use in genetic analysis such as DNA Amplifiers, Genetic Analyzers, etc.

Distributer

Natural or legal person in the supply chain who, on his own behalf, furthers the availability of a medical device to the end user

Importer

natural or legal person in the supply chain who is the first in a supply chain to make a medical device,
manufactured in another country or jurisdiction, available in the country or jurisdiction where it is to
be marketed

Manufacturer

natural or legal person with responsibility for design and/or manufacture of a medical device with the
intention of making the medical device available for use, under his name; whether or not such a medical
device is designed and/or manufactured by that person himself or on his behalf by another person(s)

Device The term "device" is used throughout the MDSAP processes. For the purpose of applying the MDSAP processes, and to accommodate nuances in the regulatory systems of the participating Regulatory Authorities, the use of the term "device" is to refer to any product that is capable of functioning as a medical device, whether or not it is packaged, labeled, or sterilized.

Supplier: Organization or individual that enters into an agreement with the acquirer or integrator for the supply of a product or service.

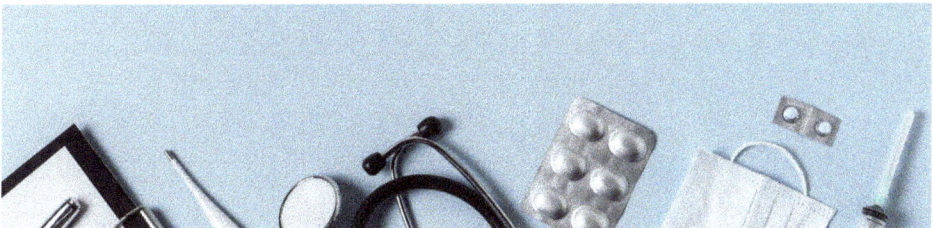

We can categorized the suppliers to:
- Critical Supplier
- Non-critical supplier

A purchased or otherwise obtained "product" or "service" is an outsourced product or service. In addition, a "supplier" is anyone that is independent from the medical device organization's quality management system. This includes a supplier that may be part of the same corporation as the medical device organization but operates under a separate quality management system from the audited medical device organization.

Critical Suppliers:

For the purposes of MDSAP, "critical suppliers" include, but are not limited to;

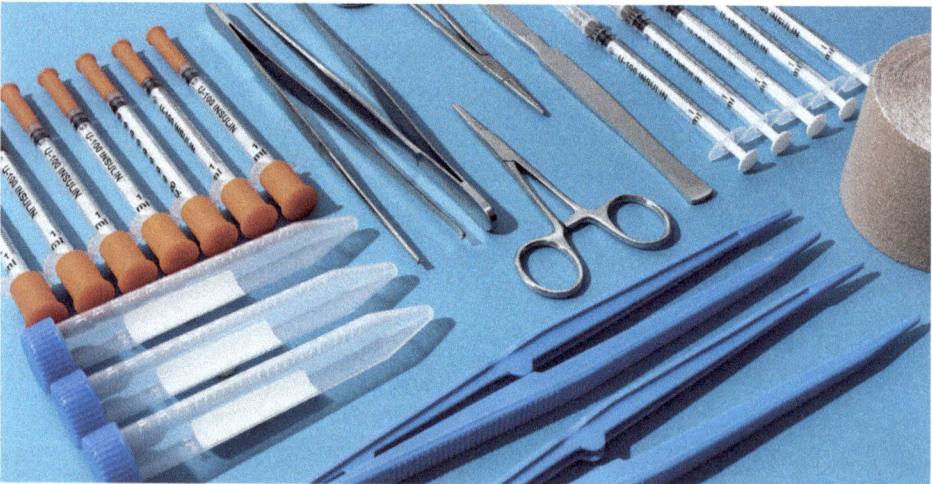

- Those entities that supply the organization with finished devices, i.e. a device, or accessory to any device, that is suitable for use or capable of functioning, whether or not it is packaged, labeled, or sterilized;
- Suppliers of products, including services, that impact design outputs that are essential for the proper functioning of the device; and
- Suppliers of products and services that require process validation.

> Not all MDSAP participating regulatory authorities require, or make use of, certification documents that relate to a medical device organization's QMS. The terms "certification" and "recertification" appear within this volumes to maintain consistency with the terminology used within ISO/IEC 17021-1:2015 Conformity assessment – Requirements for bodies providing audit and certification of management systems.

MDSAP Audit

The Medical Device Single Audit Program is based on a three (3) year audit cycle. The Initial Audit, also referred to as the "Initial Certification Audit" is a complete audit of a medical device organization's quality management system (QMS) consisting of:

Stage 1 Audit (17021-1:2015 – Cl 9.3.1.2)

Stage 2 Audit (17021-1:2015 – Cl 9.3.1.3)

The initial Audit is followed by a partial Surveillance Audit (17021-1:2015 – Cl 9.6.2.2) in each of the following two (2) years and a complete Re-audit, also referred to as a "Recertification Audit" (17021-1:2015 – Cl 9.6.3.2) in the third (3rd) year. A recertification audit may also include a Stage 1 audit if there have been significant changes to the QMS that have not been otherwise adequately assessed.

Initial Certification Audit

Initial Certification audit consists of: Stage 1 & 2

Stage 1

Documentation review, evaluation of preparedness for Stage 2 audit, etc.

A Stage 1 audit shall be conducted in accordance with Clause 9.3.1.2 of ISO/IEC 17021-1:2015 and all applicable MDSAP Audit Process tasks and regulatory requirements.

From an MDSAP perspective, the primary purposes of a Stage 1 audit are (1) to determine if QMS documentation required by ISO 13485:2016 - Clauses 4.2.1 and other applicable MDSAP documentation requirements have been adequately defined, and documented; (2) to assess the medical device organization's preparedness for a Stage 2 audit; (3) to provide a focus for planning a Stage 2 audit; and, (4) to collect information regarding the scope of the quality management system and other aspects of the medical device organization.

Portions of a Stage 1 audit (e.g. documentation review) may be performed at a site other than the site(s) of the medical device organization seeking initial certification.

The outcome of the Stage 1 audit will assist the MDSAP recognized Auditing Organization in its determination of the readiness of the medical device organization to undergo a Stage 2 audit. The Au-

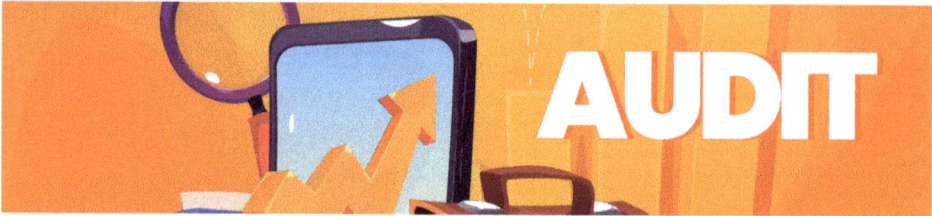

diting Organization shall determine how best to accomplish tasks of Stage 1 and Stage 2 with regards to off-site documentation and record review and on-site verifications. Hence portions of a Stage 1 audit (e.g. documentation review) may be performed at a site other than the site(s) of the medical device organization seeking initial certification. In practice it is intended that the Auditing Organization may combine elements of Stage 1 and Stage 2 to allow for a single on-site visit for the initial audit or re-audit of the medical device organization.

Stage 2

Evaluation of QMS Implementation and Effectiveness

A Stage 2 audit shall be conducted in accordance with Clause 9.3.1.3 of ISO/IEC 17021-1:2015 and using all applicable MDSAP Audit Process tasks.

The purpose of a Stage 2 audit is to determine if all applicable requirements of ISO 13485:2016 and the relevant regulatory requirements from participating regulatory authorities have been implemented. Stage 2 audit objectives shall specifically include an evaluation of:

- The effectiveness of the medical device organization's QMS incorporating the applicable regulatory requirements;
- Product/process related technologies (e.g. injection molding, sterilization);
- Adequate product technical documentation in relation to relevant regulatory requirements; and,
- The medical device organization's ability to comply with these requirements.

Surveillance Audits

(1st and 2nd Surveillance Audits):

A Surveillance Audit shall be conducted in accordance with Clause 9.6.2.2 of ISO/IEC 17021-1:2015 and clause 9.6.2 of IMDRF/MDSAP WG/N3:2016 and using applicable MDSAP Audit Process tasks. The purpose of a series of surveillance audits is to assure that all applicable requirements of ISO 13485:2016 and the relevant regulatory requirements from participating regulatory authorities are audited during the cycle of a three year audit program for the medical device organization. Surveillance audit objectives during the audit cycle shall specifically include evaluation of:

- The effectiveness of the medical device organization's QMS incorporating the applicable regulatory requirements.
- The medical device organization's ability to comply with these requirements; and
- New or changed product/process related technologies; and,
- New or amended product technical documentation in relation to relevant regulatory requirements.

In addition, surveillance audits shall include a review of issues related to medical device safety and effectiveness since the last audit such as complaints, problem reports, vigilance reports, and recalls/field corrections/advisory notices.

Re-audit (Recertification Audits)

A Re-audit (Recertification Audit) shall be conducted in accordance with Clause 9.6.3 of ISO/IEC 17021-1:2015 and using all applicable MDSAP Audit Process tasks. The purpose of a re-audit is

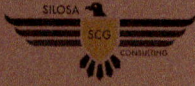

Sample Q

as a P

ISO 13

MI

Your Company Quality Plan

Your Company Organizational Chart

Your Produc

Vision

Mi

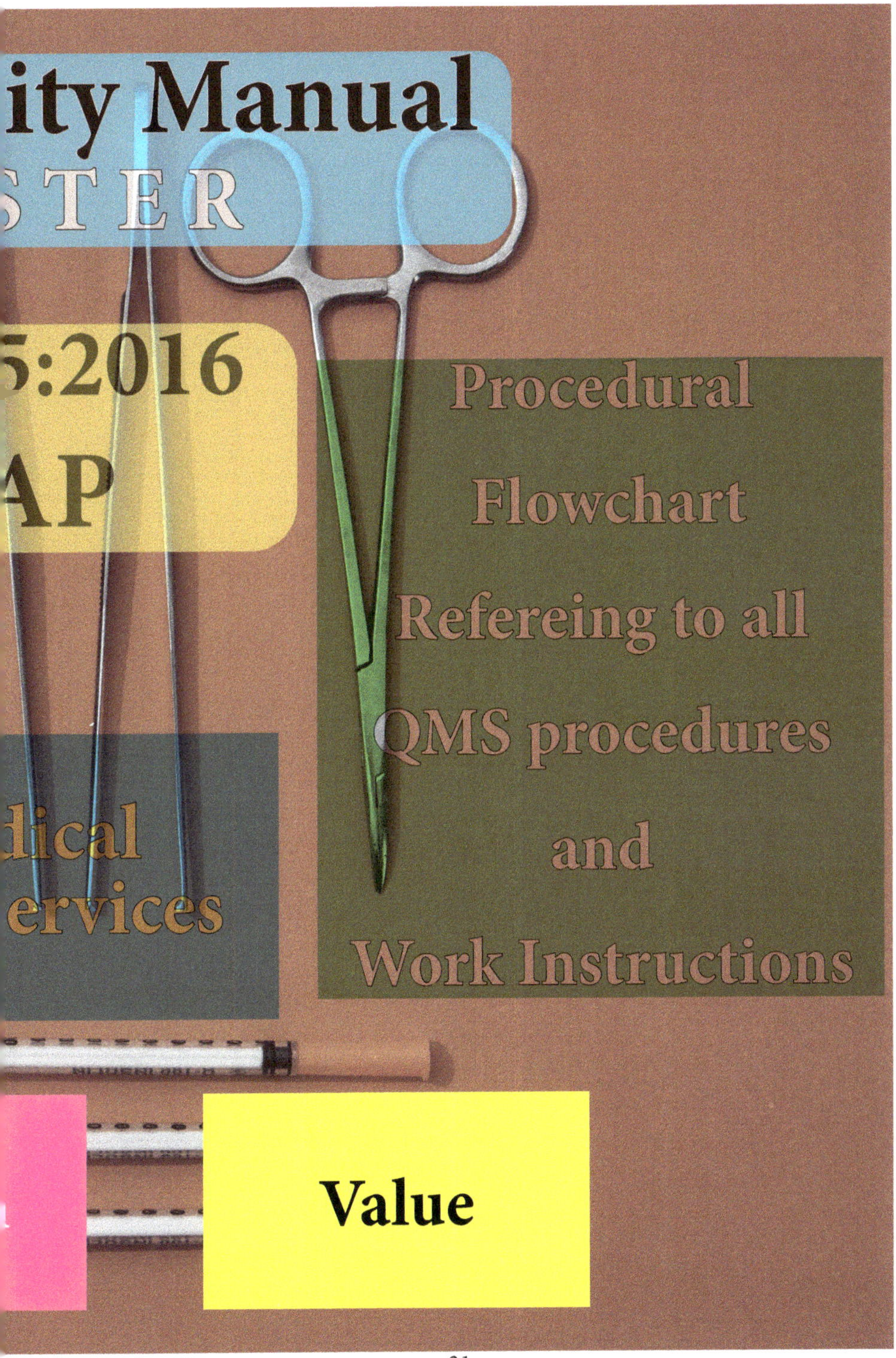

ity Manual

STER

5:2016

AP

dical
ervices

Procedural

Flowchart

Refereing to all

QMS procedures

and

Work Instructions

Value

to confirm the continued relevance, applicability and suitability of the medical device organization's QMS (as a whole), to satisfy all applicable requirements of ISO 13485:2016 and the relevant regulatory requirements from participating regulatory authorities, with respect to the scope of certification. Recertification audit objectives shall specifically include evaluation of:
- the effectiveness of the medical device organization's QMS incorporating the applicable regulatory requirements
- product/process related technologies (e.g. injection molding, sterilization)
- adequate product technical documentation in relation to relevant regulatory requirements
- the medical device organization's continued fulfillment of these requirements.

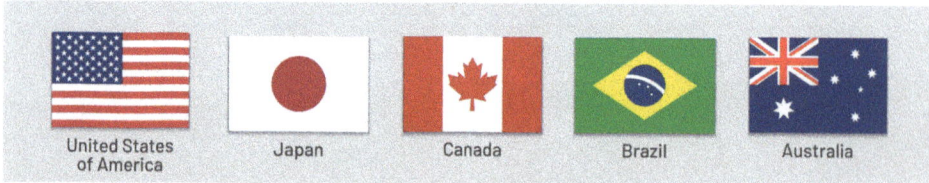

| United States of America | Japan | Canada | Brazil | Australia |

Audits Conducted by Regulatory Authorities

Audits may also be conducted by MDSAP participating regulatory authorities at any time and for a range of reasons including (1) "For Cause" due to information obtained by the regulatory authority, (2) as follow up to the findings of a previous audit, and (3) to confirm the effective implementation of MDSAP requirements by MDSAP recognized auditing organizations.

The purpose of audits conducted by regulatory authorities is to ensure appropriate oversight of a recognized MDSAP Auditing Organization's audit activities, as an alternative means of assessing medical device organizations that have been identified as undertaking high risk manufacturing processes and have not been adequately audited, where sufficient detail regarding audited processes has not been included in an audit report, or where there is a history of low compliance with QMS or regulatory requirements.

MDSAP
ISO 13485 Requirements &

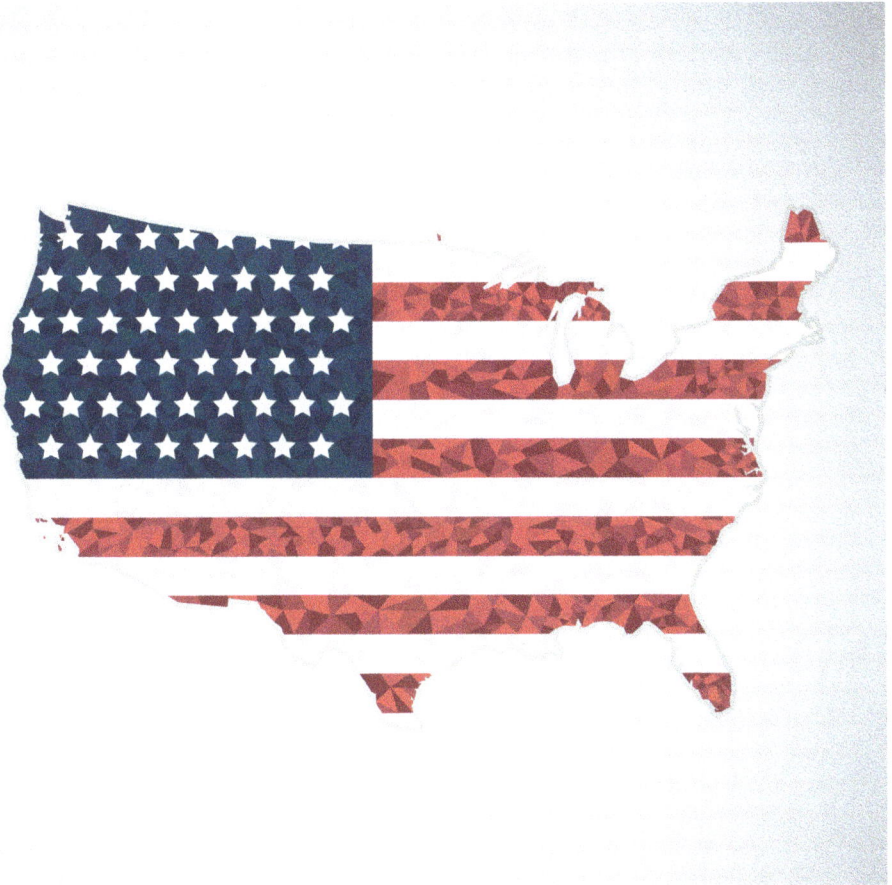

Management

The intent of the Management Process is to provide adequate resources for device design, manufacturing, quality assurance, distribution, installation, and servicing activities; to assure the quality management system is functioning properly and effectively; and to monitor the quality management system and make necessary adjustments. A quality management system that has been implemented effectively and is monitored to identify and address existing and potential problems is more likely to produce medical devices that function as intended.

The management representative is responsible for ensuring that the requirements of the quality management system have been effectively defined, documented, implemented, and maintained. Prior to the audit of a process, it may be helpful to interview the management representative (or designee) to obtain an overview of the process and a feel for management's knowledge and understanding of the process.

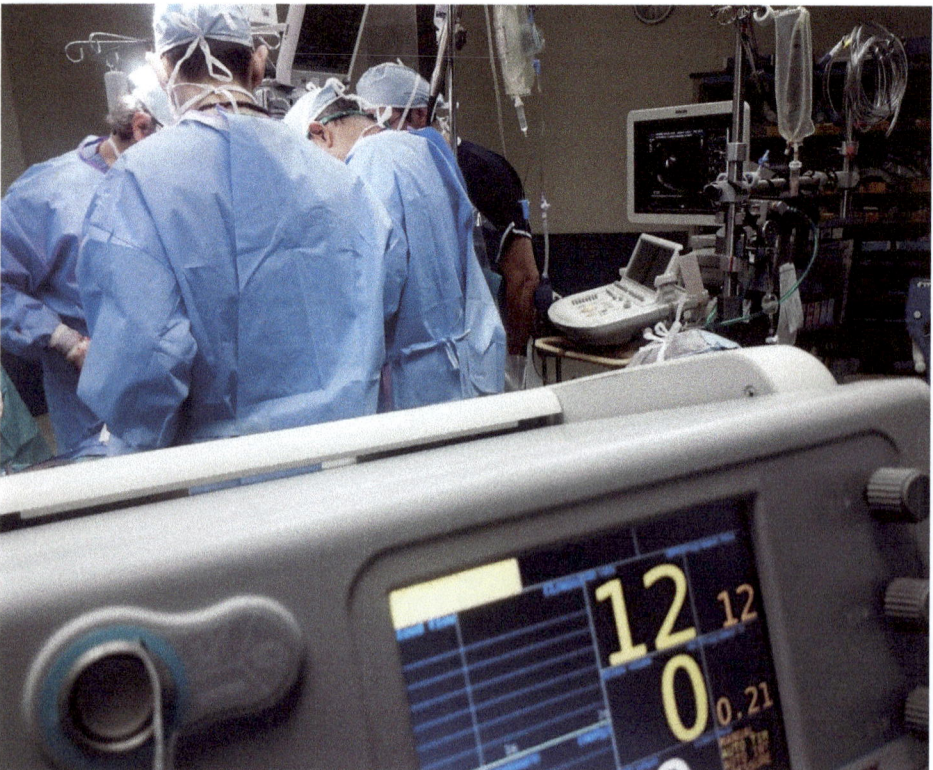

Clause and Regulation:
ISO 13485:2016: 4.1.1, 4.1.2, 4.1.3, 4.2.2, 4.1.4, 5.4.2;
FDA: 21 CFR 820.20, FDA: 21 CFR 820.20(b),
FDA: 21CFR 820.20(a), FDA: 21 CFR 820.40, 820.180
FDA: 21 CFR 820.20(a), 820.5,

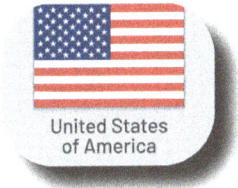

United States
of America

Verify that electronic records and documents have backups
[21 CFR 820.180].
Confirm that the medical device organization has defined, documented, and implemented procedures for control of quality management system documents and records. Evidence that these controls
are effective can be ascertained through the audit of the other quality management system processes. For example, evidence that the
document controls process is ineffective might be the observation
of obsolete procedures being used or required records being unavail-
able.
Ensure at least one copy of obsolete controlled documents is maintained. Confirm that top management has shown commitment to the
risk management process by ensuring the provision of adequate resources and the assignment of qualified personnel for risk management activities. Risk-based decisions occur throughout the various
quality management system processes. Top management is responsible for defining and documenting the policy for determining criteria
for risk acceptability. Additionally, ensure top management reviews
the suitability of the risk management process. This review may be
part of the management review. Previously unidentified risks discov-
ered during production and post-production of the medical device
may indicate a need to improve the risk management process. Each
medical device organization must decide how much risk is acceptable.

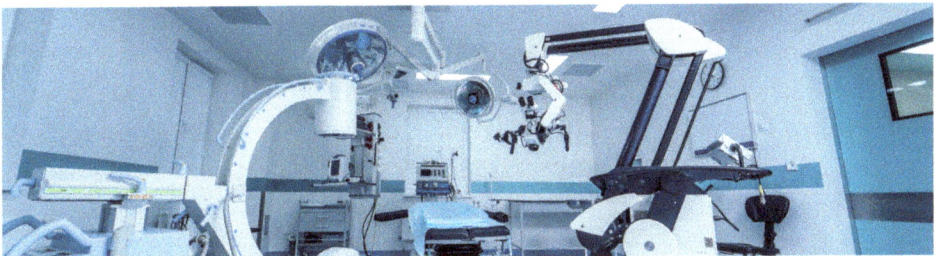

Device Marketing Authorization and Facility Registration

The Device Marketing Authorization and Facility Registration process may be audited as a linkage from the Management process and/or the Design and Development process.

ISO: ISO 13485:2016: 4.1.1, 4.2.1, 5.2, 7.2.1, 7.2.3

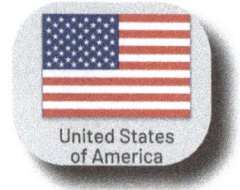

United States
of America

21 CFR 807 - Establishment Registration and Device Listing for Manufacturers and Initial Importers of Devices.

Establishment means a place of business under one management at one general physical location at which a device is manufactured, assembled, or otherwise processed.

Owner or operator means the corporation, subsidiary, affiliated company, partnership, or proprietor directly responsible for the activities of the registering establishment.

Owner or operator must register the establishment and submit listing information to Food and Drug Administration (FDA) for those devices in commercial distribution, regardless of classification.

The registration and listing requirements must pertain to any person who:

- Initiates or develops specifications for a device that is to be manufactured by a second party for commercial distribution by the person initiating specifications

- Manufactures for commercial distribution a device either for itself or for another person; regardless of whether the manufacturer places the device into commercial distribution or returns the device to the customer

- Repackages or relabels a device

-Acts as an initial importer, except that initial importers may fulfill their listing obligation for any device for which they did not initiate or develop the specifications for the device or repackage or relabel the device by submitting the name and address of the manufacturer

- Manufactures components or accessories which are ready to be used for any intended health-related purpose and are packaged or

labeled for commercial distribution for such purpose
- Sterilizes or otherwise makes a device for or on behalf of a specification developer or any other person
- Acts as a complaint file establishment
- Is a device establishment located in a foreign trade zone.

21 CFR 807.81- Premarket Notification:
Each person who is required to register his establishment pursuant to 807.20 must submit a premarket notification submission to the Food and Drug Administration at least 90 days before he proposes to begin the introduction or delivery for introduction into interstate commerce for commercial distribution of a device intended for human use which meets any of the following criteria:
- The device is being introduced into commercial distribution for the first time; that is, the device is not of the same type as, or is not substantially equivalent to, (i) a device in commercial distribution before May 28, 1976, or (ii) a device introduced for commercial distribution after May 28, 1976, that has subsequently been reclassified into class I or II.
- The device is being introduced into commercial distribution for the first time by a person required to register.

21 CFR 814 – Premarket Approval
A Premarket approval is required for any FDA class III device that was not on the market (introduced or delivered for introduction into commerce for commercial distribution) before May 28, 1976, and is not substantially equivalent to a device on the market before May 28, 1976, or to a device first marketed on, or after that date, which has been classified into class I or class II.

21 CFR 807 - Establishment Registration and Device Listing for Manufacturers and Initial Importers of Devices.
Update the device listing information during each June and December or, at its discretion, at the time the change occurs. Conditions that require updating and information to be submitted for each of these updates are as follows:
- If an owner or operator introduces into commercial distribution a device identified with a classification name not currently listed by the owner or operator
- If an owner or operator discontinues commercial distribution of all

devices in the same device class

Update registration if changes in individual ownership, corporate or partnership structure, or location of at the time of annual registration, or by letter if the changes occur at other times. This information must be submitted within 30 days of such changes. Changes in the names of officers and/or directors of the corporation(s) must be filed with the establishment's official correspondent and must be provided to the Food and Drug Administration upon receipt of a written request for this information.

21 CFR 807.81- Premarket Notification:

A new complete 510(k) application is required for changes or modifications to an existing device, where the modifications could significantly affect the safety or effectiveness of the device, or the device is to be marketed for a new or different indication. All changes in indications for use require the submission of a 510(k).

Examples of modifications that may require a 510(k) submission include, but are not limited to, the following:

- Sterilization method
- Structural material
- Manufacturing method
- Operating parameters or conditions for use
- Patient or user safety features
- Sterile barrier packaging material
- Stability or expiration claims
- Design.

21 CFR 814.39 – PMA Supplements

After FDA's approval of a PMA, an applicant shall submit a PMA supplement for review and approval by FDA before making a change affecting the safety or effectiveness of the device for which the applicant has an approved PMA. While the burden for determining whether a supplement is required is primarily on the PMA holder, changes for which an applicant shall submit a PMA supplement include, but are not limited to, the following types of changes if they affect the safety or effectiveness of the device:

- New indications for use of the device
- Labeling changes
- The use of a different facility or establishment to manufacture,

process, or package the device
- Changes in sterilization procedures
- Changes in packaging
- Changes in the performance or design specifications, circuits, components, ingredients, principle of operation, or physical layout of the device
- Extension of the expiration date of the device based on data obtained under a new or revised stability or sterility testing protocol that has not been approved by FDA
- An applicant may make a change in a device after FDA's approval of a PMA for the device without submitting a PMA supplement if the change does not affect the device's safety or effectiveness and the change is reported to FDA in post approval periodic reports required as a condition to approval of the device, e.g., an editorial change in labeling which does not affect the safety or effectiveness of the device.

Clause and Regulation
ISO: ISO 13485:2016: 4.2.1, 8.1, 8.2.1, 8.2.6, 8.5
FDA: 21 CFR 820.100(a), 21 CFR 820.100 (a)(2)

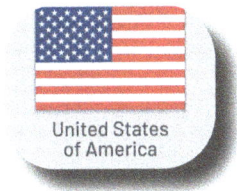

United States
of America

Measurement, Analysis and Improvement

One of the most important activities in the quality management system is the identification of existing and potential causes of product and quality problems. Such causes must be identified so that appropriate and effective corrective or preventive actions can take place. These activities are carried out under the Measurement, Analysis and Improvement process.

Verify procedures ensure that information related to quality problems or nonconforming product is disseminated to those directly responsible for assuring the quality of such product or the prevention of problems [21 CFR 820.100(a)(6)].

Confirm procedures provide for the submission of relevant information on identified quality problems, as well as corrective and preventive actions, for management review
[21 CFR 820.100(a)(7)].

Medical Device Adverse Events and Advisory Notices Reporting
The Medical Device Adverse Events and Advisory Notices Reporting process may be audited as a linkage from the Measurement, Analysis and Improvement process.

Clause and Regulation
ISO: ISO 13485:2016: 4.2.1, 7.2.3, 8.2.2, 8.2.2, 8.2.3, 8.3.3

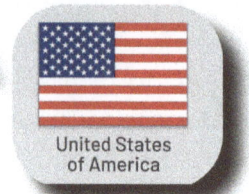

United States
of America

21 CFR 803: Medical Device Reporting
Determine whether the manufacturer has developed a process for reporting to FDA incidents involving device-related deaths, serious injuries, and reportable malfunctions that occur within and outside the United States if the same or similar device is marketed to the United States.
Confirm that the manufacturer has developed, maintained, and implemented written medical device reporting (MDR) procedures for the following:
- Internal processes that provide for:
- Timely and effective identification, communication, and evaluation of events that may be subject to MDR requirements
- A standardized review process or procedure for determining when an event meets the criteria for reporting
- Timely transmission of complete medical device reports to FDA
- Documentation and recordkeeping requirements for:
- Information that was evaluated to determine if an event was reportable;
- All medical device reports and information submitted to FDA
- Processes that ensure access to information that facilitates timely follow-up and audit.
Verify that reports are made within 30 calendar days after the day that the manufacturer receives or otherwise becomes aware of information, from any source, that reasonably suggests that a device that is marketed may have caused or contributed to a death or serious injury:
- Confirm the manufacturer's MDR files contain the following:
- Information (or references to information) related to the ad-

verse event, including all documentation of deliberations and decision-making processes used to determine if a device- related death, serious injury, or malfunction was or was not reportable to FDA
- Copies of all MDR forms and other information related to the event submitted to FDA.

If a device has malfunctioned and this device or a similar device that is marketed would be likely to cause or contribute to a death or serious injury, if the malfunction were to recur, quarterly summary reporting is acceptable for most device product codes.

If the manufacturer maintains MDR event files as part of the complaint file, ensure that the manufacturer has prominently identified these records as MDR reportable events. FDA will not consider a submitted MDR report to comply with 21 CFR 803 unless the manufacturer evaluates an event in accordance with the quality management system requirements. Confirm that the manufacturer has documented and maintained in the MDR event files an explanation of why the manufacturer did not submit or could not obtain any information required by 21 CFR 803, as well as the results of the evaluation of each event.

Compare the information submitted on the individual medical device report to the information contained in the associated complaint and confirm the medical device report contains all information related to the event that is reasonably known to the manufacturer.

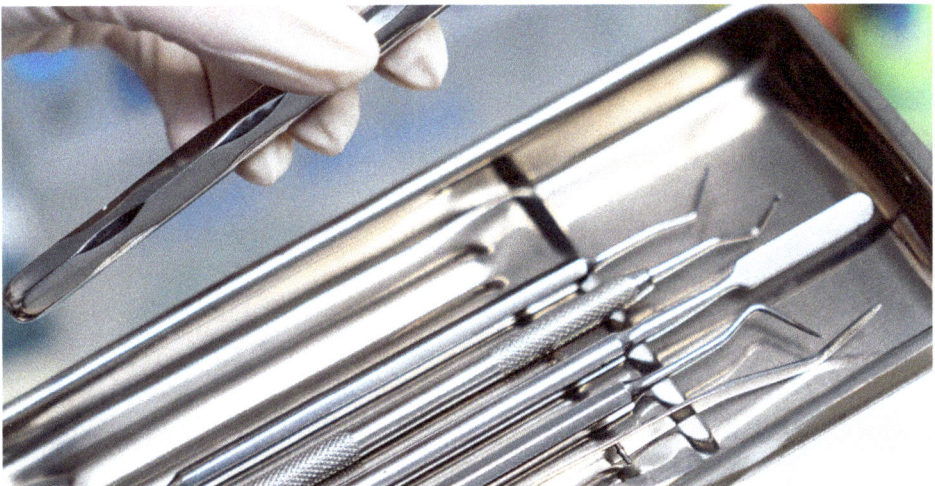

Design and Development

The purpose of the Design and Development process is to control the design of a medical device and to assure that the device meets user needs, intended use, and its specified requirements. Attention to design and development planning, identifying design inputs, developing design outputs, verifying that design outputs meet design inputs, validating the design, controlling design changes, reviewing design results, transferring the design to production, and compiling the appropriate records will help a medical device organization assure that resulting designs will meet user needs, intended uses, and requirements. Review of the Design and Development process will also provide an opportunity to evaluate how the medical device organization has utilized risk management activities to ensure design inputs are comprehensive and meet user needs, to confirm that risk control measures that were planned have been implemented in the design, and to verify that risk control measures are effective in controlling or reducing risk.

Clause and Regulation
ISO: ISO 13485:2016: 4.1.1, 4.2.1, 7.1, 7.3.10, 7.3.2
FDA: 21 CFR 820.30(a), 820.30(b), 820.30(j)

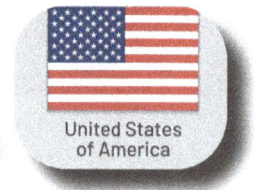

United States
of America

Verify that the design input procedures contain a mechanism for addressing incomplete, ambiguous, or conflicting requirements [21 CFR 820.30(c)].

Confirm that the manufacturer has identified the possible hazards associated with the device in both normal and fault conditions. The risks associated with the hazards, including those resulting from user error, should be calculated in both normal and fault conditions.
If any risk is judged to be unacceptable, it should be reduced to acceptable levels by the appropriate means. Ensure changes to the device to eliminate or minimize hazards do not introduce new hazards [21 CFR 820.30(g); preamble comment 83].

Production and Service Controls

The purpose of the Production and Service Controls process is to manufacture products that meet specifications. Developing processes that are adequate to produce devices that meet specifications, validating (or fully verifying the results of) those processes, and monitoring and controlling those processes are all steps that help assure the result will be devices that meet specified requirements. After completing the audit of the medical device organization's Production and Service Controls process, the audit team will return to the Management process to make a final decision of whether top management ensures that an adequate and effective quality management system has been established and maintained at the medical device organization.

Clause and Regulation
ISO: ISO 13485:2016: 7.1, 7.2.1, 7.5.1, 8.2.5, 8.2.6
FDA: 21 CFR 801, 820.30(b), 820.20(a), 820.30(h), 820.70(a), 830

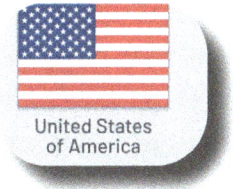

United States
of America

Confirm that the medical device organization has determined the applicability of unique device identifier requirements per 21 CFR 801 and 21 CFR 830, has obtained the unique device identifiers from an FDA-accredited UDI-issuing agency, and the required data elements have been entered in the Global Unique Device Identification Database (GUDID) [21 CFR 801, 830].

Process validation is required for sterilization, aseptic processing, injection molding, and welding
[21 CFR 820.75; preamble comment 143].

If a control number is required for traceability, confirm that a control number is on, or accompanies the device throughout distribution [21 CFR 820.120(e)].

Confirm that labeling is stored in a manner that provides proper identification and prevents mix-ups. Verify labeling and packaging operations are controlled to prevent labeling mix-ups [21 CFR 820.120(c) and (d)].

Verify that the label and labeling used for each production unit, lot, or batch are documented in the batch record, as well as any control numbers used [21 CFR 820.120(e), 820.184(e)].

Reviewing a validation

During review of a validation study, determine when applicable whether:

- The instruments used to generate the data were properly calibrated and maintained
- Predetermined product and process specifications were established
- Sampling plans used to collect test samples are based on a statistically valid rationale
- Data demonstrates predetermined specifications were met consistently
- Process tolerance limits were challenged
- Process equipment was properly installed, adjusted, and maintained
- Process monitoring instruments were properly calibrated and maintained
- Changes to the validated process were appropriately challenged (if applicable)
- Process operators were appropriately qualified.

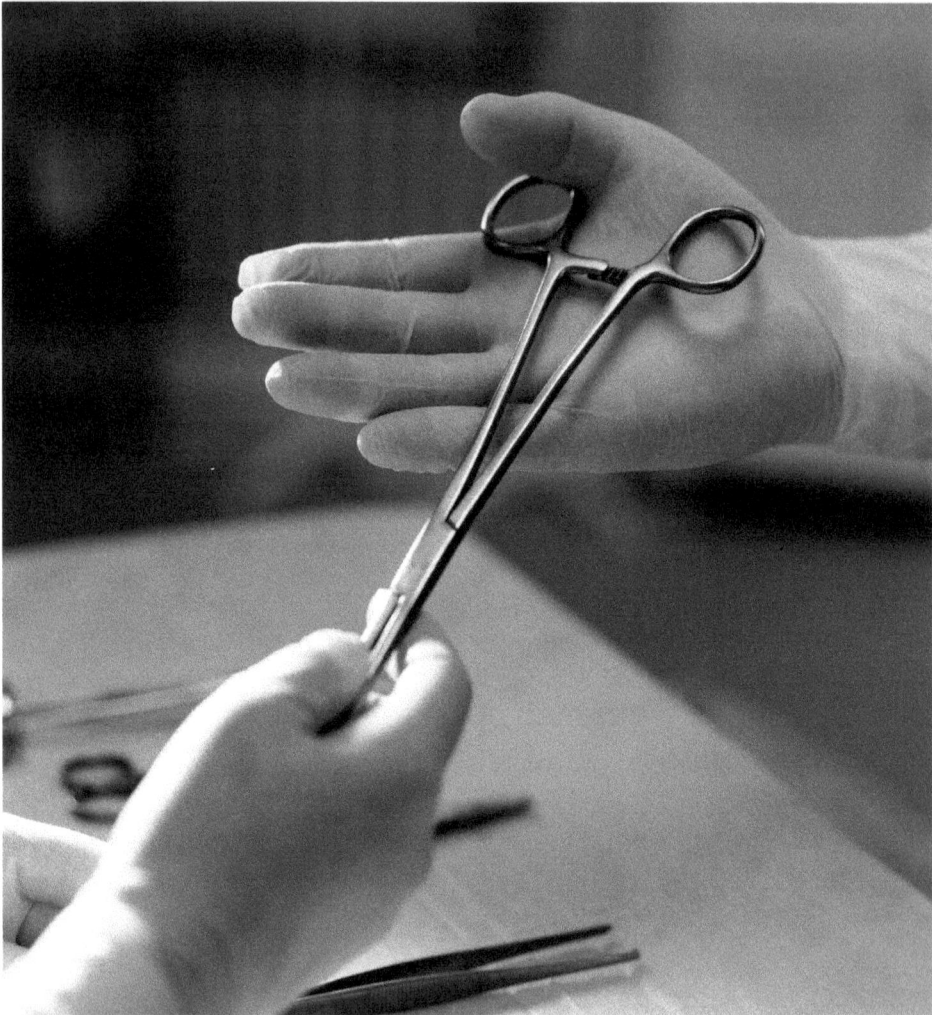

Purchasing

The intent of the Purchasing process is to ensure that purchased, sub-contracted, or otherwise received products and services conform to specified requirements. The medical device organization is expected to establish and maintain documented controls for planning and performing purchasing activities. The controls necessary depend on the effect of the product on the quality, safety, and effectiveness of the finished device. Effective purchasing processes incorporate purchasing requirements and specifications, the selection of acceptable suppliers based on the capability of the suppliers to provide acceptable product, the performance of necessary acceptance activities, and maintenance of the required quality records.

The management representative is responsible for ensuring that the requirements of the quality management system have been effectively defined, documented, implemented, and maintained. Prior to the audit of a process, it may be helpful to interview the management representative to obtain an overview of the process and a feel for management's knowledge and understanding of the process.

Clause and Regulation
ISO: ISO: ISO 13485:2016: 4.1.2, 4.1.3, 4.1.5, 7.1,
7.4.1, 7.4.2, 7.4.3

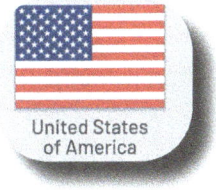

United States
of America

Planning

In planning product realization, the medical device organization must determine as appropriate the quality objectives and requirements for the purchased products, the processes, documents, and resources specific to the purchased products, the criteria for purchased product acceptance, and the required verification, monitoring, inspection, and test activities specific to the purchased products. Planning of product realization often begins in the design and development of the product, including the translation of the design into production specifications. The translation of the design into production specifications includes the establishment of specified requirements for purchased product.

Quality objectives

Quality objectives are typically expressed as a measurable target or goal. The planning of product realization should include consideration of how the purchased product, the criteria for purchased product acceptance, and the required verification, monitoring, inspection, and test activities specific to the purchased product will achieve the quality objectives.

- Some examples of QOB include:
- Number of complaints -v- number of parts shipped
- On-time delivery %
- Supplier parts rejected
- Comparison of internal audit findings -v- external audit findings
- Achieving a certain accuracy if you're developing product - based software
- Annual Post-market surveillance
- Auditing our system for regulatory compliance

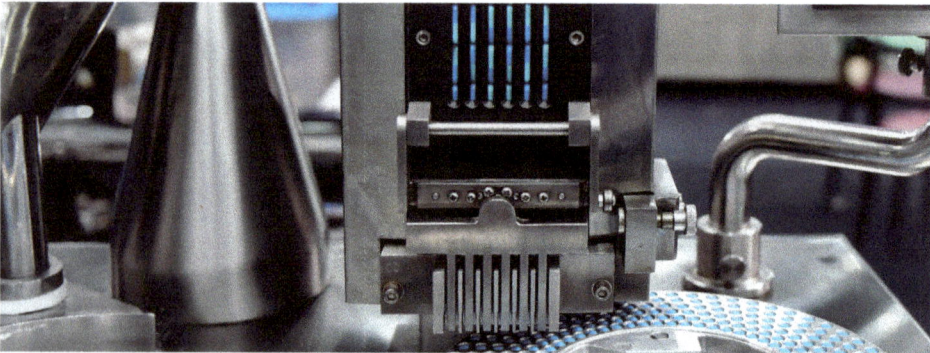

Some managers believe that the reward for hard work should be a paycheck. That's sort of like telling your children that they get to eat for doing something you're proud of. Employees are not children, but you are responsible for developing them into more valuable employees so that they can be promoted. If there is no incentive, your team will not be engaged. Therefore, pick a reward that is proportional to the bottom-line impact. Five percent of the bottom-line impact is what I like to target, but you would be amazed at how effective a few small rewards at each milestone can be. If you have trouble getting management approval for rewards, remind your boss of the bottom-line impact and link the rewards closely to the impact.

United States
of America

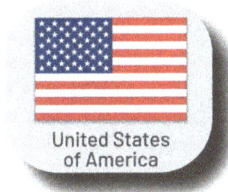

MDSAP
Audit Checklist

	REQUIREMENTS
4 Quality management system	
4.1 General requirements	
	Has the organization:
	a) identified the processes needed for the quality management system and their application throughout the organization (see 1.2)?
	b) determined the sequence and interaction of these processes?
	c) determined criteria and methods needed to ensure that both the operation and control of these processes are effective?
	d) ensured the availability of resources and information necessary to support the operation and monitoring of their processes?
	e) monitored, measured, and analyzed these processes
	f) implemented actions necessary to achieve planned results and maintain the effectiveness of these processes?
	Does the organization manage these processes in accordance with the requirements of this International Standard?
	Where an organization chooses to outsource any process that affects product conformity with requirements, does the organization ensure control over such processes?
	Is the control of such outsourced processes identified within the quality management system? (see 8.5.1)
4.2.1 General	

Doc. Reference	Adequate?	Stage I (clauses marked *)	Stage II
	Y/N	Initial›s	Initial›s

	REQUIREMENTS
	Does the quality management system documentation include:
	a) documented statements of a quality policy and quality objectives?
	b) a quality manual?
	c) documented procedures required by this international standard?
	d) documents needed by the organization to ensure the effective planning, operation and control of its processes?
	e) records required by this International Standard (see 4.2.4)?
	f) any other documentation specified by national or regional regulations?
	Has the organization established and maintained a file for each type or model of medical device either containing or identifying documents defining product specifications and quality system requirements (see 4.2.3)?
	Do these documents define the complete manufacturing process and, if applicable, installation and servicing?
Canada	Verify that the manufacturer maintains distribution records that contain sufficient information to permit complete and rapid withdrawal of the medical device from the market [CMDR 53-52].
	Verify that distribution records of a device are retained by the manufacturer in a manner that will allow for timely retrieval, for the longer of (a) the projected useful life of the device; and (b) two years after the date the device was shipped [CMDR 56-55].

Doc. Reference	Adequate?	Stage I (clauses marked *)	Stage II

	REQUIREMENTS
US	Verify that the manufacturer maintains distribution records which include or refer to the location of the name and address of the initial consignee, the identification and quantity of devices shipped; and any control numbers used [21 CFR 820.160(b)].
EU	Does the file contain or refer to the location of objective evidence establishing the safety and effectiveness of the device as required by Annex 1 of the MDD? (MDD Annex I)

4.2.2 Quality manual	
	Has the organization established and maintained a quality manual that includes:
	a) the scope of the quality management system, including details of and justification for any exclusion and/or non-application (see 1.2)?
	b) the documented procedures established for the quality management system, or reference to them?
	c) a description of the interaction between the processes of the quality management system?
	Does the quality manual outline the structure of the documentation used in the quality management system?
US	Confirm the establishment is registered with FDA and devices marketed to the United States are listed. Confirm the manufacturer has submitted a pre-market notification or approval (as applicable) to FDA prior to marketing the device in the United States [21 CFR 807].
EU	Are the applicable sections of the Medical Device Directive (MDD) included in the specified requirements throughout the documented quality system? Interpretation: A statement only indicating compliance/conformity with the relevant international or EU regulatory requirements is not acceptable.

4.2.3 Control of documents

Doc. Reference	Adequate?	Stage I (clauses marked *)	Stage II

	REQUIREMENTS
	Are documents required by the quality management system controlled?
	Is a documented procedure established to define the controls needed:
	a) To review and approve documents for adequacy prior to issue?
	b) To review and update as necessary and re-approve documents?
	c) To ensure that changes and the current revision status of documents are identified?
	d) To ensure that relevant versions of applicable documents are available at points of use?
	e) To ensure the documents remain legible and readily identifiable?
	f) To ensure that documents of external origin are identified and their distribution controlled?
	g) To prevent the unintended use of obsolete documents and to apply suitable identification to them if they are retained for any purpose?
	Does the organization ensure that changes to documents are reviewed and approved either by the original approving function or another designated function which has access to pertinent background information upon which to base its decisions?
	Does the organization define the period for which at least one copy of obsolete controlled documents shall be retained?
	Does this period ensure that documents to which medical devices have been manufactured and tested are available for at least the lifetime of the medical device as defined by the organization, but not less than the retention period of any resulting record (see 4.2.4), or as specified by relevant regulatory requirements?

Doc. Reference	Adequate?	Stage I (clauses marked *)	Stage II

	REQUIREMENTS
US	Confirm that approved changes to documents are communicated to the appropriate personnel in a timely manner [21 CFR 820.40(b)].
4.2.4 Control of quality records	
	Are records established and maintained to provide evidence of conformity to requirements and of the effective operation of the quality management system?
	Do records remain legible, readily identifiable and retrievable?
	Has a documented procedure been established to define the controls needed for the identification, storage, protection, retrieval, retention time and disposition of records?
	Does the organization retain the records for a period of time at least equivalent to the lifetime of the medical device as defined by the organization, but not less than two years from the date of product release by the organization or as specified by relevant regulatory requirements?
EU	Has the manufacturer retained for a period ending at least five years after the last product has been manufactured, the records listed in Annex II, 6.1 or Annex V, 5.1 or Annex VI, 5.1 (whichever applies)
5 Management responsibility	
5.1 Management commitment	

Doc. Reference	Adequate?	Stage I (clauses marked *)	Stage II

	REQUIREMENTS
	Has top management provided evidence of its commitment to the development and implementation of the quality management system and maintaining its effectiveness by:
	a) Communicating to the organization the importance of meeting customer as well as statutory and regulatory requirements?
	b) Establishing the quality policy?
	c) Ensuring that quality objectives are established?
	d) Conducting management reviews?
	e) Ensuring the availability of resources?
5.2 Customer focus	
	Does top management ensure that customer requirements are determined and met (see 7.2.1 and 8.2.1)?
5.3 Quality policy	
	Does top management ensure that the quality policy
	a) Is appropriate to the purpose of the organization?
	b) Includes a commitment to comply with requirements and to maintain the effectiveness of the quality management system?
	c) Provides a framework for establishing and reviewing quality objectives?
	d) Is communicated and understood within the organization?
	e) Is reviewed for continuing suitability?
5.4 Planning	
5.4.1 Quality objectives	
	Does top management ensure that quality objectives, including those needed to meet requirements for product (see 7.1a), are established at relevant functions and levels within the organization?
	Are quality objectives measurable?

Doc. Reference	Adequate?	Stage I (clauses marked *)	Stage II

	REQUIREMENTS
	Are quality objectives consistent with the quality policy?
5.4.2 Quality management system planning	
	Has top management ensured that:
	a) The planning of the quality management system is carried out in order to meet the requirements given in 4.1, as well as the quality objectives?
	b) The integrity of the quality management system is maintained when changes to the quality management system are planned and implemented?
US	Confirm the organization has established a quality plan which defines the quality practices, resources, and activities relevant to devices that are designed and manufactured (21 CFR 820.20(d))
5.5 Responsibility, authority and communication	
5.5.1 Responsibility and authority	
	Has top management ensured that responsibilities and authorities were defined, documented and communicated within the organization?
	Has top management established the interrelation of all personnel who manage, perform and verify work affecting quality, and ensured the independence and authority necessary to perform these tasks?
5.5.2 Management representative	

Doc. Reference	Adequate?	Stage I (clauses marked *)	Stage II

	REQUIREMENTS
	Has top management appointed a member of management who, irrespective of other responsibilities, has responsibility and authority that includes:
	a) Ensuring that processes needed for the quality management system are established, implemented, and maintained?
	b) Reporting to top management on the performance of the quality management system and any need for improvement (see 8.5)?
	c) Ensuring the promotion of awareness of regulatory and customer requirements throughout the organization?
5.5.3 Internal communication	
	Has top management ensured that appropriate communication processes have been established within the organization and that communication takes place regarding the effectiveness of the quality management system?
5.6 Management review	
5.6.1 General	
	Does top management review the organization's quality management system, at planned intervals, to ensure its continuing suitability, adequacy and effectiveness?
	Does this review include assessing opportunities for improvement and the need for changes to the quality management system, including the quality policy and quality objectives?
	Are records from management reviews maintained (see 4.2.4)?
5.6.2 Review input	

Doc. Reference	Adequate?	Stage I (clauses marked *)	Stage II

	REQUIREMENTS
	Does the input to management review include information on:
	a) Results of audits?
	b) Customer feedback?
	c) Process performance and product conformity?
	d) Status of preventive and corrective actions?
	e) Follow-up actions from previous management reviews?
	f) Changes that could affect the quality management system?
	g) Recommendations for improvement?
	h) New or revised regulatory requirements?
5.6.3 Review output	
	Does output from the management review include any decisions and actions related to:
	a) Improvements needed to maintain the effectiveness of the quality management system and its processes?
	b) Improvement of product related to customer requirements?
	c) Resource needs?
6 Resource management	
6.1 Provision of resources	
	Does the organization determine and provide the resources needed:
	a) To implement the quality management system and to maintain its effectiveness?
	b) To meet regulatory and customer requirements?
6.2 Human resources	
6.2.1 General	
	Are personnel performing work affecting product quality competent on the basis of appropriate education, training, skills and experience?
6.2.2 Competence, awareness and training	

Doc. Reference	Adequate?	Stage I (clauses marked *)	Stage II

	REQUIREMENTS
	Does the organization:
	a) determine the necessary competence for personnel performing work affecting product quality?
	b) Provide training or take other actions to satisfy these needs?
	c) Evaluate the effectiveness of actions taken?
	d) Ensure that its personnel are aware of the relevance and importance of their activities and how they contribute to the achievement of the quality objectives?
	e) Maintain appropriate records of education, training, skills and experience (see 4.2.4)?
US	Verify that resources include the assignment of trained personnel to meet the requirements of 21 CFR Part 820, including management, performance of work, assessment activities, and internal quality audits [21 CFR 820.20(b)(2)].
6.3 Infrastructure	
	Does the organization determine, provide and maintain the infrastructure needed to achieve conformity to product requirements?
	Infrastructure includes, as applicable:
	a) Buildings, workspace and associated utilities
	b) Process equipment, both hardware and software
	c) Supporting services such as transport or communication
	Does the organization establish documented requirements for maintenance activities, including their frequency, when such activities or lack thereof can affect product quality?
	Are records of such maintenance maintained (see 4.2.4)?
	Has the organization determined and does it manage the work environment needed to achieve conformity to product requirements?

Doc. Reference	Adequate?	Stage I (clauses marked *)	Stage II

	REQUIREMENTS
	a) Has the organization established documented requirements for health, cleanliness and clothing of personnel if contact between such personnel and the product or work environment could adversely affect the quality of the product (see 7.5.1.2.1)?
	b) If work environment conditions can have an adverse effect on product quality, has organization established documented requirements for the work environment conditions and documented procedures or work instructions to monitor and control these work environment conditions (see 7.5.1.2.1)?
	c) Does the organization ensure that all personnel who are required to work temporarily under special environmental conditions within the work environment are appropriately trained or supervised by a trained person [see 6.2.2 b)]?
	d) If appropriate, are special arrangements established and documented for the control of contaminated or potentially contaminated product in order to prevent contamination of other product, the work environment or personnel (see 7.5.3.1)?
7 Product realization	
7.1 Planning of product realization	
	Has the organization planned and developed the processes needed for product realization?
	Is the planning of product realization consistent with the requirements of the other processes of the quality management system (see 4.1)?

Doc. Reference	Adequate?	Stage I (clauses marked *)	Stage II

	REQUIREMENTS
	In planning product realization, has the organization determined the following, as appropriate:
	a) Quality objectives and requirements for products?
	b) The need to establish processes, documents, and provide resources specific to the product?
	c) Required verification, validation, monitoring, inspection and test activities specific to the product and the criteria for product acceptance?
	d) Records needed to provide evidence that the realization processes and resulting product meet requirements (see 4.2.4)?
	Is the output of this planning in a form suitable for the organization's method of operations?
	Does the organization establish documented requirements for risk management throughout product realization and are records arising from risk management maintained (see 4.2.4)?
US	Confirm that the manufacturer has identified the possible hazards associated with the device in both normal and fault conditions. The risks associated with the hazards, including those resulting from user error, should be calculated in both normal and fault conditions. If any risk is judged to be unacceptable, it should be reduced to acceptable levels by the appropriate means. Ensure changes to the device to eliminate or minimize hazards do not introduce new hazards [21 CFR 820.30(g); preamble comment 83].
EU	Does the supplier evaluate the need for risk analysis throughout the design process and maintain records of any risk analysis performed? (MDD Annex 1)
	7.2.1 Determination of requirements related to the product

Doc. Reference	Adequate?	Stage I (clauses marked *)	Stage II

	REQUIREMENTS
	Has the organization determined:
	a) Requirements specified by the customer, including the requirements for delivery and post-delivery activities?
	b) Requirements not stated by the customer but necessary for specified or intended use, where known?
	c) Statutory and regulatory requirements related to the product?
	d) Any additional requirements determined by the organization?
EU	Vefiy that manufacturing maintains files containing or refer to the location of objective evidence establishing the safety and effectiveness of the device as required by Annex 1 of the MDD. Verify that the manufacturer followed a defined and effective process to establish and maintain a file containing documents defining product specifications and quality system requirements for each newa and existing type/modes of medical devices. Since the last audit, has the manufacturer introduced new products in the EU? Has the manufacturer followed a defined and effective process to obtain an approval from the Notified Body to CE mark a product prior to selling it in the EU? (does not apply to class I devices)

Doc. Reference	Adequate?	Stage I (clauses marked *)	Stage II

	REQUIREMENTS
USA	Verify that the firm has the appropriate marketing clearance [510(k)] or pre-market approval (PMA) if distributing the devices in the United States [21 CFR 807]. 21 CFR -807.81 When a pre-market notification is required: Each person who is required to register his establishment pursuant to 807.20 must submit a premarket notification submission to the Food and Drug Administration at least 90 days before he proposes to begin the introduction or delivery for introduction into interstate commerce for commercial distribution of a device intended for human use which meets any of the following criteria: (1) The device is being introduced into commercial distribution for the first time; that is, the device is not of the same type as, or is not substantially equivalent to, (i) a device in commercial distribution before May 1976 ,28, or (ii) a device introduced for commercial distribution after May ,28 1976, that has subsequently been reclassified into class I or II. (2) The device is being introduced into commercial distribution for the first time by a person required to register 21 CFR 814 – Premarket Approval; A Premarket approval is required for any FDA class III device that was not on the market (introduced or delivered for introduction into commerce for commercial distribution) before May ,28 1976, and is not substantially equivalent to a device on the market before May 1976 ,28, or to a device first marketed on, or after that date, which has been classified into class I or class II.
7.2.2 Review of requirements related to the product	
	Does the organization review the requirements related to the product?

Doc. Reference	Adequate?	Stage I (clauses marked *)	Stage II

	REQUIREMENTS
	Is this review conducted prior to the organization's commitment to supply a product to the customer (e.g. submission of tenders, acceptance of contracts or orders, acceptance of changes to contracts or orders)?
	Does the organization ensure that:
	a) Product requirements are defined and documented?
	b) Contract or order requirements differing from those previously expressed are resolved?
	c) The organization has the ability to meet the defined requirements?
	Are records of the results of the review and actions arising from the review maintained (see 4.2.4)?
	Where the customer provides no documented statement of requirement, are the customer requirements confirmed by the organization before acceptance?
	Where product requirements are changed, does the organization ensure that relevant documents are amended and that relevant personnel are made aware of the changed requirements?
7.2.3 Customer communication	
	Has the organization determined and implemented effective arrangements for communicating with customers in relation to:
	a) Product information?
	b) Enquiries, contracts or order handling, including amendments?
	c) Customer feedback, including customer complaints? (see 8.2.1)
	d) Advisory notices? (see 8.5.1)
7.3 Design and development	
7.3.1 Design and/or development planning	

Doc. Reference	Adequate?	Stage I (clauses marked *)	Stage II

		REQUIREMENTS
		Has the organization established documented procedures for design and development?
		Does the organization plan and control the design and development of product?
		During the design and development planning, does the organization determine:
		a) The design and development stages?
		b) The review, verification, validation and design transfer activities (see Note) that are appropriate at each design and development stage?
		c) The responsibilities and authorities for design and development?
		Does the organization manage the interfaces between different groups involved in design and development to ensure effective communication and clear assignment of responsibility?
		Is planning output documented, and updated as appropriate, as the design and development progresses? (See 4.2.3)
7.3.2 Design and development inputs		
		Have inputs relating to product requirements been determined and records maintained (see 4.2.4)?
		Do these inputs include:
		a) Functional, performance and safety requirements, according to the intended use?
		b) Applicable statutory and regulatory requirements?
		c) Where applicable, information derived from previous similar designs?
		d) Other requirements essential for design and development?
		e) Output(s) of risk management (see 7.1)?
		Are these inputs reviewed for adequacy and approved?

Doc. Reference	Adequate?	Stage I (clauses marked *)	Stage II

		REQUIREMENTS
		Are requirements complete, unambiguous and not in conflict with each other?
	US	Verify that the design input procedures contain a mechanism for addressing incomplete, ambiguous, or conflicting requirements [21 CFR 820.30(c)].
	7.3.3 Design and development outputs	
		Are the outputs of design and development provided in a form that enables verification against the design and development input, and is it approved prior to release?
		Do design and development outputs:
		a) meet the input requirements for design and development?
		b) Provide appropriate information for purchasing, production and for service provision?
		c) Contain or reference product acceptance criteria?
		d) Specify the characteristics of the product that are essential for its safe and proper use?
		Are records of the design and development outputs maintained (see 4.2.4)?
	7.3.4 Design and development review	
		At suitable stages, are systematic reviews of design and development performed in accordance with planned arrangements (see 7.3.1):
		a) To evaluate the ability of the results of design and development to meet requirements?
		b) To identify any problems and propose necessary actions?
		Do participants in such reviews include representatives of functions concerned with the design and development stage(s) being reviewed, as well as other specialist personnel (see 5.5.1 and 6.2.1)?
	US	Are records of the results of the reviews and any necessary actions maintained (see 4.2.4)?

Doc. Reference	Adequate?	Stage I (clauses marked *)	Stage II

	REQUIREMENTS
US	Verify that procedures ensure that participants include representatives of all functions concerned with the design stage being reviewed and an individual(s) who does not have direct responsibility for the design stage being reviewed, as well as any specialists needed [21 CFR 820.30(e)].
EU	Does the supplier evaluate the need for risk analysis throughout the design process and maintain records of any risk analysis performed? (MDD Annex 1)
7.3.5 Design and development verification	
	Is verification performed in accordance with planned arrangements (see 7.3.1) to ensure that the design and development outputs have met the design and development input requirements?
	Are records of the results of the verification and any necessary actions maintained?
7.3.6 Design and development validation	
	Is design and development validation performed in accordance with planned arrangements (see 7.3.1) to ensure that the resulting product is capable of meeting the requirements for the specified application or intended use?
	Is validation completed prior to the delivery or implementation of the product (see Note 1)?
	Are records of the results of validation and any necessary actions maintained (see 4.2.4)?
	As part of design and development validation, does the organization perform clinical evaluations and/or evaluation of performance of the medical device, as required by national or regional regulations (see Note 2)?

Doc. Reference	Adequate?	Stage I (clauses marked *)	Stage II

	REQUIREMENTS
US	Verify that design validation has been performed on initial production units, lots, or batches, or their equivalents. When equivalent devices are used in the final validation, the manufacturer must document in detail how the device was manufactured and how the device is similar to and possibly different from initial production. When there are differences, the manufacturer must justify why design validation results are valid for the production units, lots, or batches. Verify that design validation includes testing of production units under actual or simulated use conditions [21 CFR 820.30(g)].
7.3.7 Control of design and development changes	
	Are design and development changes identified and records maintained?
	Are changes reviewed, verified, and validated, as appropriate, and approved before implementation?
	Does the review of design and development changes include evaluation of the effect of the changes on constituent parts and product already delivered?
	Are records of the results of the review of changes and any necessary actions maintained?
US	Verify that the firm obtained a new 510(k) or supplement to the pre-market approval if required [21 CFR 807].
EU	Do documented procedures identify the need to report essential changes to the Notified Body, (MDD Annex II, V, VI, 3.4)
7.4 Purchasing	
7.4.1 Purchasing process	
	Has the organization established documented procedures to ensure that purchased product conforms to specified purchase requirements?

Doc. Reference	Adequate?	Stage I (clauses marked *)	Stage II

	REQUIREMENTS
	Is the type and extent of control applied to the supplier and the purchased product dependent upon the effect of the purchased product on subsequent product realization or the final product?
	Does the organization evaluate and select suppliers based on their ability to supply product in accordance with the organization's requirements?
	Have criteria for selection, evaluation and re-evaluation been established?
	Are records of the results of evaluation and any necessary actions arising from the evaluation maintained (see 4.2.4)?
	Does purchasing information describe the product to be purchased, including where appropriate:
	a) Requirements for approval of product, procedures, processes and equipment?
	b) Requirements for qualification of personnel?
	c) Quality management system requirements?
	Does the organization ensure the adequacy of specified purchase requirements prior to their communication to the supplier?
	To the extent required for traceability given in 7.5.3.2, does the organization maintain relevant purchasing information, i.e. documents (see 4.2.3) and records (see 4.2.4)?
7.4.3 Verification of purchased product	
	Has the organization established and implemented the inspection or other activities necessary for ensuring that purchased product meets specified purchase requirements?
	Where the organization or its customer intends to perform verification at the supplier's premises, does the organization state the intended verification arrangements and method of product release in the purchasing information?
	Are records of the verification maintained (see 4.2.4)?

Doc. Reference	Adequate?	Stage I (clauses marked *)	Stage II

	REQUIREMENTS

7.5 Production and service provision	
7.5.1 Control of production and service provision	
7.5.1.1 General Requirements	
	Does the organization plan and carry out production and service provision under controlled conditions?
	Do the controlled conditions include, as applicable:
	a) The availability of information that describes the characteristics of the product?
	b) The availability of documented procedures, documented requirements, work instructions, reference materials and reference measurement procedures as necessary?
	c) The use of suitable equipment?
	d) The availability and use of monitoring and measuring devices?
	e) The implementation of monitoring and measurement?
	f) The implementation of release, delivery and post-delivery activities?
	g) The implementation of defined operations for labeling and packaging?
	Does the organization establish and maintain a record (see 4.2.4) for each batch of medical devices that provides traceability to the extent specified in 7.5.3 and identifies the amount manufactured and amount approved for distribution?
	Is the batch record verified and approved?

Doc. Reference	Adequate?	Stage I (clauses marked *)	Stage II

	REQUIREMENTS
US	Verify that labeling is not released for storage or use until a designated individual has examined the labeling for accuracy. The release, including the date and signature of the individual performing the examination must be documented in the device history record (i.e. batch record) [21 CFR 820.120(b)]. Confirm that labeling is stored in a manner that provides proper identification and prevents mix-ups. Verify that labeling and packaging operations are controlled to prevent labeling mix-ups [21 CFR 820.120(c) and (d)]. Verify that the label and labeling used for each production unit, lot, or batch are documented in the batch record, as well as any control numbers used [21 CFR 820.120(e), 820.184(e)].

7.5.1.2 Control of production and service provision — Specific requiremen

7.5.1.2.1 Cleanliness of product and contamination control

	Does the organization establish documented requirements for cleanliness of product if:
	a) Product is cleaned by the organization prior to sterilization and/or its use, or
	b) Product is supplied non-sterile to be subjected to a cleaning process prior to sterilization and/or its use, or
	c) Product is supplied to be used non-sterile and its cleanliness is of significance in use, or
	d) Process agents are to be removed from product during manufacture?
	If product is cleaned in accordance with a) or b) above, the requirements contained in 6.4 a) and 6.4 b) do not apply prior to the cleaning process.

7.5.1.2.2 Installation activities

Doc. Reference	Adequate?	Stage I (clauses marked *)	Stage II

	REQUIREMENTS
	If appropriate, does the organization establish documented requirements which contain acceptance criteria for installing and verifying the installation of the medical device?
	If the agreed customer requirements allow installation to be performed other than by the organization or its authorized agent, does the organization provide documented requirements for installation and verification?
	Are records of installation and verification performed by the organization or its authorized agent maintained (see 4.2.4)?
7.5.1.2.3 Servicing activities	
	If servicing is a specified requirement, does the organization establish documented procedures, work instructions and reference materials and reference measurement procedures, as necessary, for performing servicing activities and verifying that they meet the specified requirements?
	Are records of servicing activities carried out by the organization maintained (see 4.2.4)?
US	Verify that each manufacturer who receives a service report that represents an event that must be reported to FDA as a medical device report automatically considers the report a complaint [21 CFR 820.200(c)]. Confirm that service reports are documented and include the name of the device serviced, any device identification(s) and control number(s) used, and the date of service [21 CFR 820.200(d)].
7.5.1.3 Particular requirements for sterile medical devices	
	Does the organization maintain records of the process parameters for the sterilization process which was used for each sterilization batch (see 4.2.4)?
	Are sterilization records traceable to each production batch of medical devices (see 7.5.1.1)?
7.5.2 Validation of processes for production and service provision	

Doc. Reference	Adequate?	Stage I (clauses marked *)	Stage II

	REQUIREMENTS
	7.5.2.1 General requirements
	Does the organization validate any processes for production and service provision where the resulting output cannot be verified by subsequent monitoring or measurement? (this includes any processes where deficiencies become apparent only after the product is in use or the service has been delivered)
	Does validation demonstrate the ability of the processes to achieve planned results?
	Has the organization established arrangements for these processes including, as applicable:
	a) Defined criteria for review and approval of the processes?
	b) Approval of equipment and qualification of personnel?
	c) Use of specific methods and procedures?
	d) Requirements for records (see 4.2.4)?
	e) Re-validation?
	Has the organization established documented procedures for the validation of the application of computer software (and changes to such software and/or its application) for production and service provision that affect the ability of the product to conform to specified requirements?
	Are such software applications validated prior to initial use?
	Are records of validation maintained (see 4.2.4)?
US	Process validation is required for sterilization, aseptic processing, injection molding, and welding [21 CFR 820.75; preamble comment 143].
US	Confirm that the validation activities and results, including the date and signature of the individual approving the validation and where appropriate the major equipment validated, have been documented [21 CFR 820.75(a)].
	7.5.2.2 Particular requirements for sterile medical devices

Doc. Reference	Adequate?	Stage I (clauses marked *)	Stage II

	REQUIREMENTS
	Has the organization established documented procedures for the validation of sterilization processes?
	Are sterilization processes validated prior to initial use?
	Are records of validation of each sterilization process maintained (see 4.2.4)?
7.5.3 Identification and traceability	
7.5.3.1 Identification	
	Does the organization identify the product by suitable means throughout product realization and does the organization establish documented procedures for such product identification?
	Has the organization established documented procedures to ensure that medical devices returned to the organization are identified and distinguished from conforming product [see 6.4 d)]?
7.5.3.2 Traceability	
7.5.3.2.1 General	
	Has the organization established documented procedures for traceability?
	Do such procedures define the extent of product traceability and the records required (see 8.3 ,4.2.4 and 8.5)?
	Does the organization control and record the unique identification of the product, where traceability is a requirement (see 4.2.4)?
US	If a control number is required for traceability, confirm that such control number is on or accompanies the device throughout distribution [21 CFR 820.120(e)].

Doc. Reference	Adequate?	Stage I (clauses marked *)	Stage II

	REQUIREMENTS
EU	Does the manufacturer have procedures identifying the requirements of labeling and instructions for use as defined in MDD, Annex 1 point 13, and is regulations for CE marking included in these procedures. (MDD 3, Article 17 and Annex 12).
	Are language requirements defined in procedures for the information identified in MDD, Annex 1point 13 for the applicable markets.
7.5.3.2.2 Particular requirements for active implantable medical devices an		
	In defining the records required for traceability, does the organization include records of all components, materials and work environment conditions, if these could cause the medical device not to satisfy its specified requirements?
	Does the organization require that its agents or distributors maintain records of the distribution of medical devices to allow traceability and that such records be available for inspection?
	Are records of the name and address of the shipping package consignee maintained (see 4.2.4)?
US	Verify that the manufacturer has implemented a tracking system for devices for which the manufacturer has received a tracking order from FDA. The tracking system must ensure the manufacturer is able to track the device to the end-user. The manufacturer must conduct periodic audits of the tracking system [21 CFR 821].
7.5.3.3 Status identification		
	Does the organization identify the product status with respect to monitoring and measurement requirements?
	Is the identification of product status maintained throughout production, storage, installation and servicing of the product to ensure that only product that has passed the required inspections and tests (or released under an authorized concession) is dispatched, used or installed?

Doc. Reference	Adequate?	Stage I (clauses marked *)	Stage II

medical devices

	REQUIREMENTS
7.5.4 Customer property	
	Does the organization exercise care with customer property while it is under the organization's control or being used by the organization?
	Does the organization identify, verify, protect and safeguard customer property provided for use or incorporation into the product?
	If any customer property is lost, damaged, or otherwise found to be unsuitable for use, is this reported to the customer and are records maintained (see 4.2.4)?
7.5.5 Preservation of product	
	Has the organization established documented procedures or documented work instructions for preserving the conformity of product during internal processing and delivery to the intended destination?
	Does this preservation include identification, handling, packaging, storage and protection, and also apply to the constituent parts of a product?
	Has the organization established documented procedures or documented work instructions for the control of product with a limited shelf-life or requiring special storage conditions?
	Are such special storage conditions controlled and recorded (see 4.2.4)?

Doc. Reference	Adequate?	Stage I (clauses marked *)	Stage II

	REQUIREMENTS
US	Confirm that the manufacturer established and maintains procedures that describe the methods for authorizing receipt from and dispatch to storage areas and stock rooms [21 CFR 150(b)]. Verify that the manufacturer established and maintains procedures for control and distribution of finished devices to ensure that only those devices approved for release are distributed and that purchase orders are reviewed to ensure ambiguities and errors are resolved before devices are released for distribution [21 CFR 820.160(a)].
7.6 Control of monitoring and measuring devices	
	Does the organization determine monitoring and measuring to be undertaken and the monitoring and measuring devices needed to provide evidence of conformity of product to determined requirements (guide reference 7.2.1)?
	Has the organization established documented procedures to ensure that monitoring and measurement can be carried out and are carried out in a manner that is consistent with the monitoring and measurement requirements?
	Where necessary to ensure valid results, is measuring equipment:
	a) Calibrated or verified at specified intervals, or prior to use, against measurement standards traceable to international or national measurement standards; where no such standards exist, is the basis used for calibration or verification recorded?
	b) Adjusted or re-adjusted as necessary?
	c) Identified to enable the calibration status to be determined?
	d) Safeguarded from adjustments that would invalidate the measurement result?
	e) Protected from damage and deterioration during handling, maintenance and storage?

Doc. Reference	Adequate?	Stage I (clauses marked *)	Stage II

	REQUIREMENTS
	Does the organization assess and record the validity of the previous measuring results when the equipment is found not to conform to requirements?
	Does the organization take appropriate action on the equipment and any product affected?
	Are records of the results of calibration and verification maintained (see 4.2.4)?
	When used in the monitoring and measurement of specified requirements, is the ability of computer software to satisfy the intended application confirmed prior to initial use and reconfirmed as necessary ?
8 Measurement, analysis and improvement	
8.1 General	
	Does the organization plan and implement the monitoring, measurement, analysis and improvement processes needed:
	a) To demonstrate conformity of the product?
	b) To ensure conformity of the quality management system?
	c) To maintain the effectiveness of the quality management system?
	Does this include determination of applicable methods, including statistical techniques, and the extent of their use?
US	Where appropriate, verify the organization has established and maintained procedures for identifying valid statistical techniques required for establishing, controlling , and verifying the acceptability of process capability and product characteristics [21 CFR 820.250(a)].
8.2 Monitoring and measurement	
8.2.1 Feedback	
	As one of the measurements of the performance of the quality management system, does the organization monitor information relating to whether the organization has met customer requirements?

Doc. Reference	Adequate?	Stage I (clauses marked *)	Stage II

		REQUIREMENTS
		Have the methods for obtaining and using this information been determined?
		Has the organization established a documented procedure for a feedback system [see 7.2.3 c)] to provide early warning of quality problems and for input into the corrective and preventive action processes (see 8.5.2 and 8.5.3)?
		If national or regional regulations require the organization to gain experience from the post-production phase, does the review of this experience form part of the feedback system (see 8.5.1)?
	Canada	Verify that the manufacturer maintains records of reported problems related to the performance characteristics or safety of a device, including any consumer complaints received by the manufacturer after the device was first sold in Canada, and all actions taken by the manufacturer in response to the problems referred to in t hecomplaints [CMDR Section 57]. Verify that the manufacturer has established and implemented documented procedures that will enable it to carry out an effective and timely investigation of the problems reports through the customer complaints, andto carry out an effective and timely recall of the device [CMDR Section 58].
	Japan	Confirm that the personnel operating the Registered Manufacturing Site has determined and implemented effective arrangements for communicating with the Japanese Marketing Authorization Holder in relation to customer feedback, including customer complaints, and advisory notices [MHLW MO29 :169].

Doc. Reference	Adequate?	Stage I (clauses marked *)	Stage II

	REQUIREMENTS
US	Verify procedures have been defined, documented, and implemented for receiving, reviewing, and evaluating complaints by a formally designated unit. Procedures must ensure that: (1) All complaints are processed in a uniform and timely manner (2) Oral complaints are documented upon receipt (3) Complaints are evaluated to determine whether the complaint represents an event which is required to be reported to FDA
	Each manufacturer must review and evaluate all complaints to determine whether an investigation is necessary. When no investigation is made, the manufacturer must maintain a record that includes the reason no investigation was made and the name of the individual responsible for the decision not to investigate. Any complaint of the failure of the device, labeling, or packaging to meet any of its specifications must be reviewed, evaluated, and investigated, unless such investigation has already been made for a similar complaint and another investigation is not necessary. Any complaint that represents an event which must be reported to FDA must be promptly reviewed, evaluated, and investigated by a designated individual(s) and must be maintained in a separate portion of the complaint files or otherwise clearly identified.
	When the manufacturer's formally designated unit is located at a site separate from the manufacturing establishment, the investigated complaint(s) and the record(s) of investigation must be reasonably accessible to the manufacturing establishment [21 CFR 820.198].

Doc. Reference	Adequate?	Stage I (clauses marked *)	Stage II

	REQUIREMENTS
8.2.2 Internal audit	
	Does the organization conduct internal audits at planned intervals to determine whether the quality management system
	a) Conforms to the planned arrangements (see 7.1), to the requirements of this International Standard and to the quality management system requirements established by the organization?
	b) Is effectively implemented and maintained?
	Is an audit programme planned, taking into consideration the status and importance of the processes and areas to be audited, as well as the results of previous audits?
	Are the audit criteria, scope, frequency and methods defined?
	Does selection of auditors and conduct of audits ensure objectivity and impartiality of the audit process (e.g. auditors shall not audit their own work)?
	Are the responsibilities and requirements for planning and conducting audits, and for reporting results and maintaining records (see 4.2.4) defined in a documented procedure?
	Does management responsible for the area being audited ensure that actions are taken without undue delay to eliminate detected nonconformities and their causes?
	Do follow-up activities include the verification of the actions taken and the reporting of verification results? (see 8.5.2)
US	Verify that resources include the assignment of trained personnel to meet the requirements of 21 CFR Part 820, including management, performance of work, assessment activities, and internal quality audits [21 CFR 820.20(b)(2)].
8.2.3 Measurement and monitoring of processes	

Doc. Reference	Adequate?	Stage I (clauses marked *)	Stage II

	REQUIREMENTS
	Does the organization apply suitable methods for monitoring and, where applicable, measurement of the quality management system processes?
	Do these methods demonstrate the ability of the processes to achieve planned results?
	When planned results are not achieved, is correction and corrective action taken, as appropriate, to ensure conformity of the product?
US	Verify that the manufacturer has established and maintains procedures for identifying valid statistical techniques required for establishing, controlling and verifying the acceptability of process capability and product characteristics, where appropriate [21 CFR 820.250(a)].
8.2.4 Monitoring and measurement of product	
8.2.4.1 General requirements	
	Does the organization monitor and measure the characteristics of the product to verify that product requirements have been met?
	Is this carried out at appropriate stages of the product realization process in accordance with the planned arrangements (see 7.1) and documented procedures (see 7.5.1.1)?
	Is evidence of conformity with the acceptance criteria maintained?
	Do records indicate the person(s) authorizing release of the product (see 4.2.4)?
	Does the organization ensure that product release and service delivery do not proceed until the planned arrangements (see 7.1) have been satisfactorily completed?

Doc. Reference	Adequate?	Stage I (clauses marked *)	Stage II

	REQUIREMENTS
US	Verify that the manufacturer establishes and maintains procedures to ensure that sampling methods are adequate for their intended use and ensure that when changes occur, the sampling plans are reviewed [21 CFR 820.250(b)].
8.2.4.2 Particular requirement for active implantable medical devices and i	
	Does the organization record (see 4.2.4) the identity of personnel performing any inspection or testing?
8.3 Control of nonconforming product	
	Does the organization ensure that product which does not conform to product requirements is identified and controlled to prevent its unintended use or delivery?
	Are the controls and related responsibilities and authorities for dealing with nonconforming product defined in a documented procedure?
	Does the organization deal with nonconforming product by one or more of the following ways?
	a) By taking action to eliminate the detected nonconformity
	b) By authorizing its use, release or acceptance under concession
	c) By taking action to preclude its original intended use or application
	Does the organization ensure that nonconforming product is accepted by concession only if regulatory requirements are met?
	Are records of the identity of the person(s) authorizing the concession maintained (see 4.2.4)?
	Are records of the nature of nonconformities and any subsequent actions taken, including concessions obtained maintained (see 4.2.4)?
	When nonconforming product is corrected, is it subject to re-verification to demonstrate conformity to the requirements?

Doc. Reference	Adequate?	Stage I (clauses marked *)	Stage II

edical devices

	REQUIREMENTS
	When nonconforming product is detected after delivery or use has started, does the organization take action appropriate to the effects, or potential effects, of the nonconformity?
	If product needs to be reworked (one or more times), does the organization document the rework process in a work instruction that has undergone the same authorization and approval procedure as the original work instruction?
	Prior to authorization and approval of the work instruction, is a determination of any adverse effect of the rework upon product made and documented (see 4.2.3 and 7.5.1)?
US	Confirm that the evaluation of non-conforming product includes a determination of the need for an investigation and notification of the persons or organizations responsible for the nonconformance. The evaluation and any investigation must be documented [21 CFR 820.90(a)].
8.4 Analysis of data	
	Does the organization establish documented procedures to determine, collect and analyse appropriate data to demonstrate the suitability and effectiveness of the quality management system and to evaluate if improvement of the effectiveness of the quality management system can be made?
	Does this include data generated as a result of monitoring and measurement and from other relevant sources?
	Does the analysis of data provide information relating to:
	a) Feedback (see 8.2.1)?
	b) Conformity to product requirements? (See 7.2.1)
	c) Characteristics and trends of processes and products including opportunities for preventive action?
	d) Suppliers?
	Are records of the results of the analysis of data maintained (see 4.2.4)?

Doc. Reference	Adequate?	Stage I (clauses marked *)	Stage II

	REQUIREMENTS
	8.5 Improvement
	8.5.1 General
	Does the organization identify and implement any changes necessary to ensure and maintain the continued suitability and effectiveness of the quality management system through the use of the quality policy, quality objectives, audit results, analysis of data, corrective and preventive actions and management review?
	Does the organization establish documented procedures for the issue and implementation of advisory notices and are these procedures capable of being implemented at any time?
US	Verify that the manufacturer has a process in place to notify FDA in the event of actions concerning device corrections and removals and to maintain records of those corrections and removals. [21 CFR 806: Medical Devices; Reports of Corrections and Removals]
EU	Are the procedures for Vigilance reporting in conformance with MDD Annex II, V, and VI (MEDDEV 1-2.12)
	Are records of all customer complaint investigations maintained (see 4.2.4)?
	If investigation determines that the activities outside the organization contributed to the customer complaint, is relevant information exchanged between the organizations involved (see 4.1)?
	If any customer complaint is not followed by corrective and/or preventive action, is the reason authorized (see 5.5.1) and recorded (see 4.2.4)?
US	Verify that information related to quality problems or nonconforming product is disseminated to those directly responsible for assuring the quality of such product or the prevention of such problems [21 CFR 820.100(a)(6)].

Doc. Reference	Adequate?	Stage I (clauses marked *)	Stage II

	REQUIREMENTS
	If national or regional regulations require notification of adverse events that meet specific reporting criteria, does the organization establish documented procedures to such notification to regulatory authorities?
US	Determine whether the manufacturer has developed a process for reporting to FDA incidents involving device-related deaths, serious injuries, and reportable malfunctions that occur within and outside the United States if the same or similar device is marketed to the United States. Confirm that the manufacturer has developed, maintained, and implemented written medical device reporting (MDR) procedures compliant with the requirements of: [21 CFR 803: Medical Device Reporting]
EU	Are procedures for the reporting of recall to the relevant competent authority and the NB compliant? (MDD, Annex II, V, VI, 3.1)
8.5.2 Corrective action	
	Does the organization take action to eliminate the cause of nonconformities in order to prevent recurrence and are corrective actions appropriate to the effects of the nonconformities encountered?

Doc. Reference	Adequate?	Stage I (clauses marked *)	Stage II

	REQUIREMENTS
	Has a documented procedure been established to define requirements for:
	a) Reviewing nonconformities (including customer complaints)?
	b) Determining the causes of nonconformities?
	c) Evaluating the need for action to ensure that nonconformities do no recur?
	d) Determining and implementing action needed, including, if appropriate, updating documentation (see 4.2)?
	e) Recording of the results of any investigation and of action taken (see 4.2.4)?
	f) Reviewing the corrective action taken and its effectiveness?
US	Verify that procedures are in place for verifying or validating the corrective and preventive action to ensure the action is effective and does not adversely affect the finished device [21 CFR 820.100(a)(4)]. Verify procedures ensure that information related to quality problems or nonconforming product is disseminated to those directly responsible for assuring the quality of such product or the prevention of problems [21 CFR 820.100(a)(6)]. Confirm procedures provide for the submission of relevant information on identified quality problems, as well as corrective and preventive actions, for management review [21 CFR 820.100(a)(7)].
8.5.3 Preventive action	
	Does the organization determine action to eliminate the causes of potential nonconformities in order to prevent their occurrence and are preventive actions appropriate to the effects of the potential problems?

Doc. Reference	Adequate?	Stage I (clauses marked *)	Stage II

	REQUIREMENTS
	Has a documented procedure been established to define requirements for:
	a) Determining potential nonconformities and their causes?
	b) Evaluating the need for action to prevent occurrence of nonconformities?
	c) Determining and implementing action needed?
	d) Recording of the results of any investigations and of action taken (see 4.2.4)?
	e) Reviewing preventive action taken and its effectiveness?

Doc. Reference	Adequate?	Stage I (clauses marked *)	Stage II

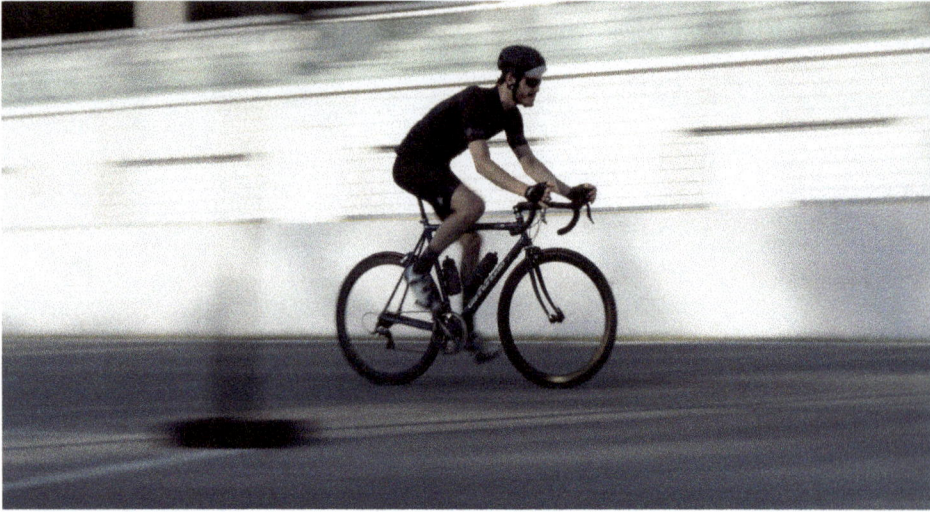

The system is working for you (the system is fully integrated along your processes and eases your operations).

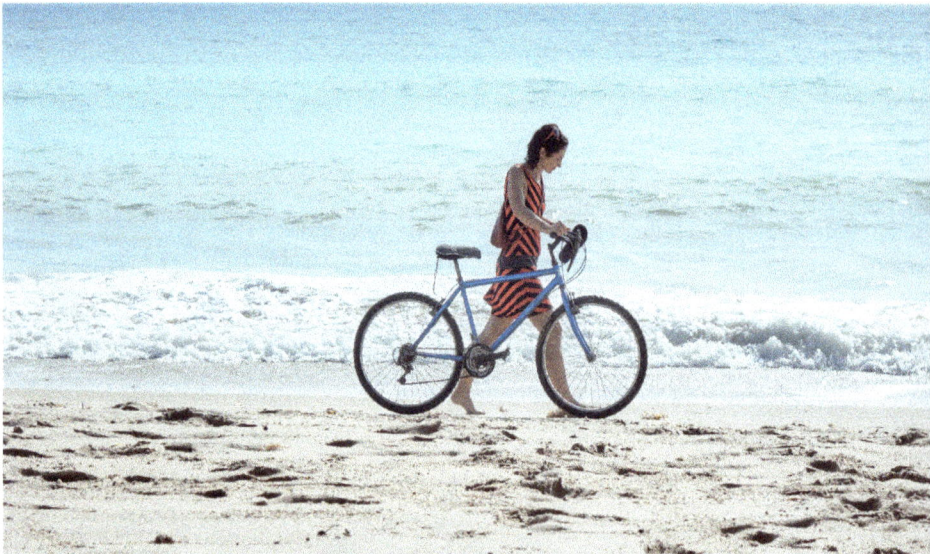

You are working for the system
(the system is beside your operations and looks as an additional burden.)

Advice for manufacturers planning certification

Firstly, you should confirm that the device(s) your company manufactures can be defined as a medical device under ISO 13485 standards; or, if you provide a medical device service, that your service is related to a product defined as a medical device. Getting ISO 13485 certification is challenging and requires commitment so, secondly, it's important that your leadership team confirms that holding the certification will add value to your company, meet its business objectives and support its strategy. While holding the full certification is not strictly necessary, as your company can still conform to and benefit from ISO 13485 standards without being externally certified, it does clearly demonstrate to all stakeholders that you comply with its requirements.

If you do want to become independently certified there are two phases; the first covers documentation, while the second implements your quality management system and audits it. You must carry out phase two within six months of completing phase one.

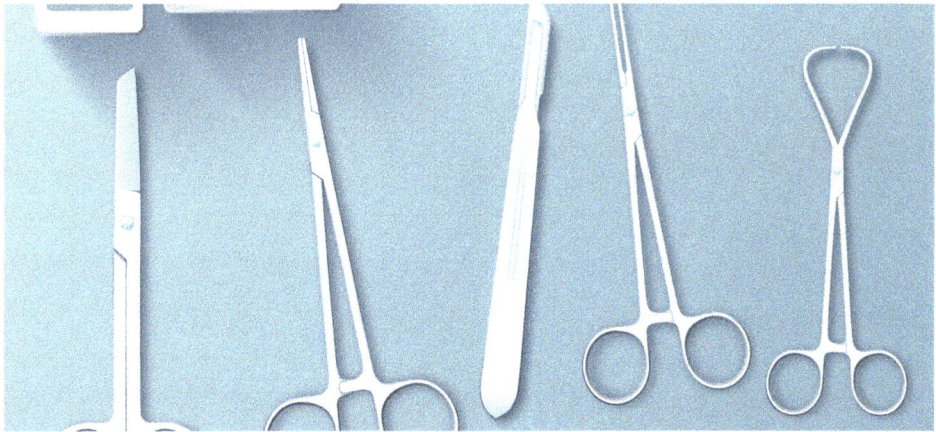

ISO 13485 certification costs

For companies who wish to be fully ISO 13485 certified, there are associated costs for external, independent certification. Although you may be under cost pressure, it's important to work with an independent auditor who will add real value to your company during the certification process. In this highly regulated industry, choose a reputable auditing company with extensive expertise rather than one that enables you to gain certification at the lowest price.

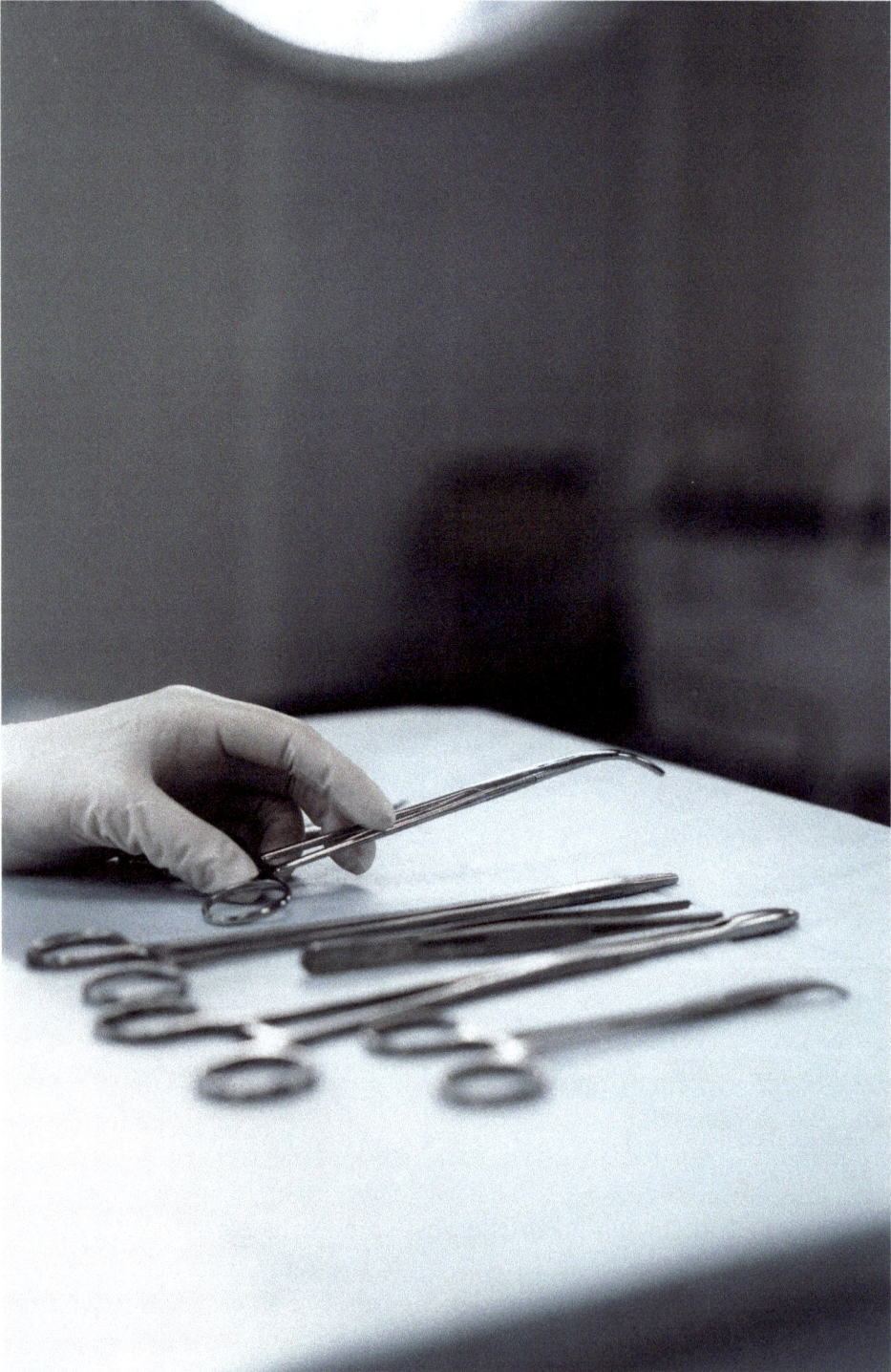

Bibliography:

Astrini, N. (2018). ISO 9001 and performance: a method review. Total Quality Management & Business Excellence, doi: 10.1080/14783363.2018.1524293.

Asadi,J, Easy ISo 13485:2016, Silosa Consulting Group, 2022

Bou-Llusar, J. C., Escrig-Tena, A. B., Roca-Puig, V., & Beltra´n-Martı´n, I. (2005). To what extent do enablers explain results in the EFQM excellence model? International Journal of Quality & Reliability Management, 22(44), 337-353.

Chatzoglou, P., Chatzoudes, D., & Kipraios, N. (2015). The impact of ISO 9000 certification on firms' financial performance. International Journal of Operations and Production Management, 35(1), 145-174. https://doi.org/10.1108/IJOPM-07-2012-0387

Definition of the terms "medical device" and "in vitro diagnostic (IVD) medical device". Global Harmonization Task Force;

Guidelines for regulatory auditing of quality systems of medical device manufacturers – Part 1: general requirements

Global Medical Devices Nomenclature System (GMDN) [website] (https://www. gmdnagency.org, accessed 2 February 2017).

FDA website address: fda.gov

Gigante, N., & Ziantoni, S. (2015). L'edizione 2015 della norma ISO 9001, 2015. Retrieved from:https://www.accredia.it/app/uploads/2015/12/6050_5_L__700_edizione_2015_della_norma_ISO_9001___Arch__Gigante__Dr__Ziantoni.pdf

ISO (2015a). ISO 9001 - Quality management systems – requirements. Geneva: International Organization for Standardization.

Role of standards in the assessment of medical devices. Global Harmonization Task Force; 2008 ISO (2018). ISO 19011 - Guidelines for auditing management systems quality management systems. Geneva: International Organization for Standardization.

ISO (2019). ISO 9000 Family - Quality Management. Retrieved from: https://www.iso.org/home.html.

Wilson, J. P., & Campbell, L. (2018). ISO 9001:2015: the evolution and convergence of quality management and knowledge management for competitive advantage. Total Quality Management and Business Excellence, pp. 1-16. https://doi.org/10.1080/ 14783363.2018.1445965

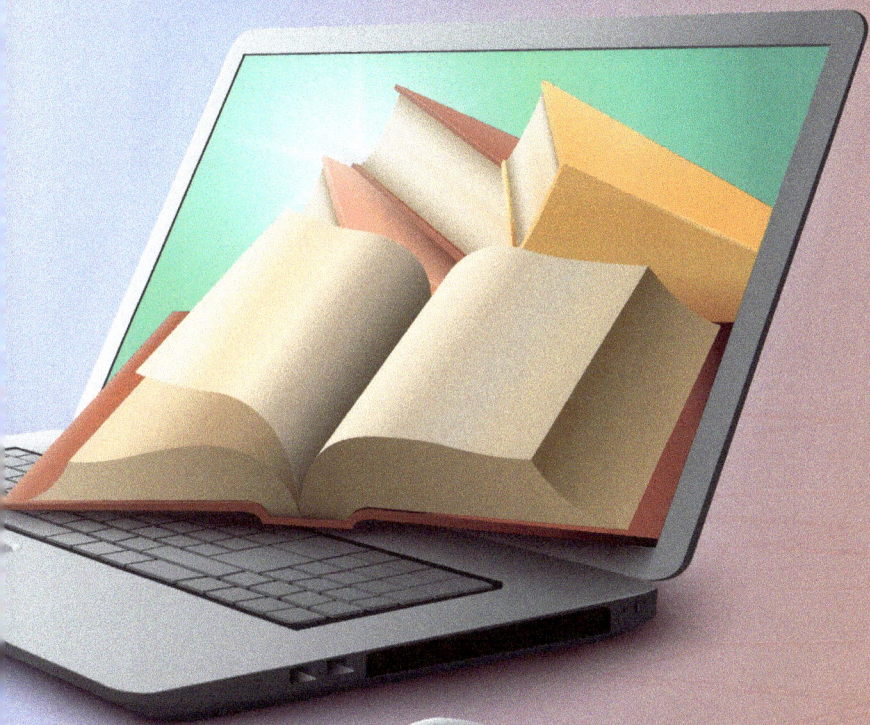

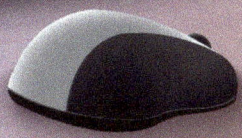

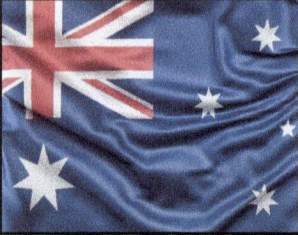	**MDSAP** **Vol.1** AUSTRALIA
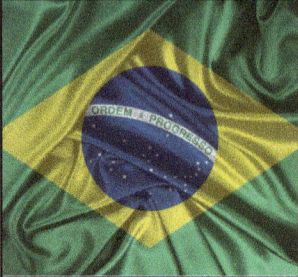	**MDSAP** **Vol.2** Brazil
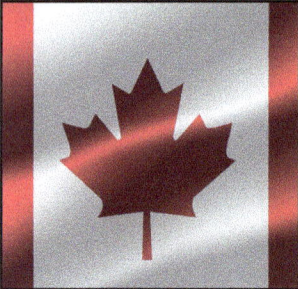	**MDSAP** **Vol.3** Canada
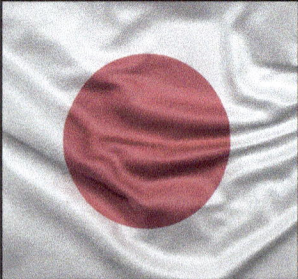	**MDSAP** **Vol.4** Japan
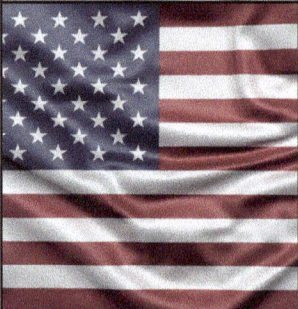	**MDSAP** **Vol.5** USA

www.ingramcontent.com/pod-product-compliance
Lightning Source LLC
Chambersburg PA
CBHW040903210326
41597CB00029B/4948